The Construction of Power and Authority in Psychiatry

This book is dedicated to all our colleagues within the survivor and user movements, and in the psychiatric disciplines in the UK, the USA, and Australia and New Zealand. We hope that this text will aid the *rapprochement* between those who provide and those who receive psychiatric services

The Construction of Power and Authority in Psychiatry

Phil Barker PhD, RN, FRCN

Professor of Psychiatric Nursing Practice,
University of Newcastle, UK

and

Chris Stevenson RMN BA(Hons), MSc(Dist), PhD

Lecturer in Psychiatric Nursing Practice,
University of Newcastle, UK

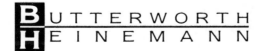

BUTTERWORTH
HEINEMANN

OXFORD   AUCKLAND   BOSTON   JOHANNESBURG   MELBOURNE   NEW DELHI

Butterworth-Heinemann
Linacre House, Jordan Hill, Oxford OX2 8DP
225 Wildwood Avenue, Woburn, MA 01801–2041
A division of Reed Educational and Professional Publishing Ltd

ℛ A member of the Reed Elsevier plc group

First published 2000

British Library Cataloguing in Publication Data
A catalogue record for this book is available from the British Library

Library of Congress Cataloguing in Publication Data
A catalogue record for this book is available from the Library of Congress

ISBN 0 7506 3839 7

Composition by Genesis Typesetting, Laser Quay, Rochester, Kent
Printed and bound in Great Britain by Biddles Ltd, www.Biddles.co.uk

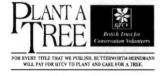

Contents

Conclusion

Contributors

Jane Andrews
Doctoral Student
University of Sunderland

Alan Armstrong
Research Associate/Doctoral
Student
Department of Psychiatry
University of Newcastle

Phil Barker
Professor of Psychiatric Nursing
Practice
Department of Psychiatry
University of Newcastle

Jim Birch
Consultant Psychiatrist
Newcastle City Health Trust

Mary Boyle
Professor of Psychology
Faculty of Science and Health
University of East London

Ron Coleman
Independent Training Consultant
Handsell Publications
Gloucester

Suman Fernando
Senior Lecturer in Mental Health
Tizard Centre
University of Kent at Canterbury

Jeffrey Fortuna
Director
The Windhorse Project
Northampton
Massachusetts
USA

Alec Jenner
Emeritus Professor of Psychiatry
University of Sheffield

Shaun Parsons
Lecturer in Psychiatric Nursing
Practice
Department of Psychiatry
University of Newcastle

Shulamit Ramon
Professor of Interprofessional
Health and Social Studies
Anglia Polytechnic University
Cambridge

Alex Reed
Lecturer Practitioner
Newcastle City Health Trust

Marius Romme
Professor in Social Psychiatry
University of Maastricht
The Netherlands

Glynnis Spriddell
Social Worker
Whitley Bay Community Mental
Health Team

Chris Stevenson
Lecturer in Psychiatric Nursing
Practice
Department of Psychiatry
University of Newcastle

Thomas Szasz
Professor of Psychiatry Emeritus
SUNY Health Science Centre
Syracuse
New York
USA

Gary Winship
Adult Psychotherapist
Psychotherapy Department
West Berkshire NHS Trust

A personal preface

Chris Stevenson

In the autumn of 1995, I was privileged to have been a member of the North Shields Family Team for more than three years. The team had come together because of a hope on the part of its members that they might relieve the dis-ease that they were feeling in relation to their previous approaches to families, which, in the main, centred on structural, strategic and early Milan schools. Our disenchantment could be summarized as concern about the them-and-us rituals of the therapy. For example, the institutionalized one-way screen, pre- and post-session conversations between the team members as experts, the prescription of tasks, and the use of paradoxical interventions. Many of the team had been following the career path of Lynn Hoffman (1981, 1985, 1990) and her narrative of personal change (Hoffman, 1992). She described her movement from being an agent of a psychiatric system based on 'secrecy, hierarchy and control' (p. 15) to a more respectful approach which acknowledged the expertise of the client about their situation (Anderson and Goolishian, 1992). The team had been exposed also to the ideas of a Norwegian doctor, Tom Andersen, and his development of the idea of a reflecting team (1987) which encourages participants in the therapy to engage in dialogue and avoid the dominance of professional monologues. My preoccupation with power, conversation and language found a conduit in co-organizing a conference that would foreground these issues. With the support of Professor Phil Barker of the University of Newcastle, Department of Psychiatry, a colleague from Newcastle City Health Trust hospital, Hazel Dunn, who agreed to join me in the project, practical support from the University of Northumbria at Newcastle and technical support from Ed Alderson and his team, the conference machine began to roll.

For me, the conference invited some 'retro'. As a student nurse I had been exposed to (and inspired by) the work in the 1950s, 1960s and 1970s of Thomas Szasz, Gregory Bateson, Ronnie Laing, David Cooper, Aaron Esterson and Erving Goffman. These figures occupied markedly different theoretical positions and yet shared the ability to make psychiatric practitioners question their 'taken-for-granted' practice, sometimes to the dismay of the psychiatric establishment. It seemed important to invite people who could speak with these voices, or with their echoes – a combination of 'elders' and 'new wave' academics and others with a perspective on psychiatric 'care'. We wanted also to confuse the boundaries around science, as the claimed power base of psychiatry, and art as different media of understanding. To this end we invited a local poet, Sean O'Brien, to compose a conference poem, which is included here. People who are in or have been in psychiatric distress embellished the physical surroundings of the conference with their paintings composed at Linskill Art Studio in North Shields.

The proposed key themes of the conference were: how power relations arise, are maintained and can be, though rarely are, problematized within psychiatry; reconsidering and deconstructing professional hegemony; how discriminatory discourse institutionalizes the disadvantage of women and people of marginalized racial origin/ethnicity; re-appraising the idea of the person as expert in relation to her/his whole lived experience; alternative ways to work respectfully with the experiences of the people who are 'veterans' of psychiatric services and who are likely to be carrying a well rehearsed diagnostic label. Underpinning these themes was an optimistic belief that psychiatry does not have to be organized in the accustomed and encultured way. Contemporary examples of work from Scandinavia, indicate that meetings involving the interested parties in psychiatric crisis can lead to avoiding admission, less psychotropic drug use and lower relapse rates (Seikkula *et al.*, 1995); and that democratic 'guest houses' can be a successful alternative to acute in-patient admission wards (Hartvikson, 1996). The recent past give us examples of Villa 21 (Cooper, 1967), Kingsley Hall, the Philadelphia Association and Arbours Association (see Laing, 1995 for a description of the establishment and anti-establishment of therapeutic houses) and the therapeutic communities established by Maxwell Jones (1952).

Perhaps the themes struck a chord in the hearts of those who were invited. From the outset, the organizers felt divinely favoured, for the 'famous names' that were contacted as potential presenters agreed to speak. A wide range of delegates were invited – service users, families of people in psychiatric distress, professionals of different disciplines – and attended, creating a rich conference milieu. In constructing the conference, we tried to be mindful of power issues. This was an event conceived of by white, middle-class professionals – academics and/or practitioners. To some extent we succeeded, in that we priced places on the basis of the ability to pay, in that service users, in common with other attendees, occupied positions of both presenters and delegates. However, power is slippery, for example, the language of a conference is not always accessible to the uninitiated, and problematic. There are no easy solutions to the issue of power relations, otherwise the conference itself would have been redundant.

The conference was held at Longhirst Hall in Northumberland, an idyllic place, which manages to combine the ancient and modern with dignity. If context does help to construct reality we had a head start in making the meeting a success. Perhaps people interested in how power is constructed are more mindful of power issues in 'everyday' relationships. Certainly, the conference was memorable because of the informal dialogue in which presenters and delegates seemed to easily engage one another. As to the formal papers and panels, the content, presented in Part One of the book, spoke and speaks for itself. The commission of this book, sought by Phil Barker, seems to me to indicate that it was an event of its time. Although the conference constructed the book in one sense, the process of bringing together the text invited the inclusion of papers produced contemporaneously, but also those of significance written before and after the event. Part Two is a treasury of complementary and critical papers.

For me, the process of the conference was almost as inspiring as the content. To hear people speak with impassioned voices, to watch an audience in rapt attention, to feel the energy generated, was its own reward. I felt myself to be in a privileged position throughout. Whilst the organizational issues were omnipresent, so were people who I would class as my heroes . . . without clay feet. That the conference was a success in and of itself is satisfying. To know that the book will 'keep alive' the spirit of Longhirst and introduce it to the collective consciousness of psychiatric professionals is, perhaps, the greatest gift of all.

REFERENCES

Andersen, T. (1987) The reflecting team: dialogue and meta-dialogue in clinical work. *Family Process*, **26**: 415–428.

Anderson, H. and Goolishian, H. (1992) The client is the expert: a non-knowing approach to therapy. In: K. Gergen and S. McNamee (eds), *Therapy as Social Construction*. London: Sage.

Cooper, D. (1967) *Psychiatry and Anti-Psychiatry*. London: Tavistock.

Hartvikson, I. (1996) Paviljongen; a guest house. A democratic alternative in the Norwegian Psychiatric Services. *Human System*, **7**: 265–274.

Hoffman, L. (1981) *Foundations of Family Therapy: A Conceptual Framework for Systems Change*. New York: Basic Books.

Hoffman, L. (1985) Beyond power and control: toward a second order family systems therapy. *Family Systems Medicine*, **3**: 381–396.

Hoffman, L. (1990) Constructing realities: an art of lenses. *Family Process*, **29**: 1–12.

Hoffman, L. (1992) A reflexive stance for family therapy. In: K. Gergen and S. McNamee (eds), *Therapy as Social Construction*. London: Sage.

Jones, M. (1952) *Social Psychiatry: A Study of Therapeutic Communities*. London: Tavistock.

Laing, A. (1995) *R.D. Laing: A Biography*. London: Peter Owen.

Seikkula, J., Aaltonen, J., Alakare, B., Haarakangas, K., Keränen, J. and Sutela, M. (1995) Treating psychosis by means of open dialogue. In: S. Friedman (ed.), *The Reflecting Team in Action*. New York: Guilford.

Acknowledgements

Context and power in family meetings (Chapter 10) is reprinted with kind permission of *Changes*.

'Manufacturing a human drama from a psychiatric crisis: crisis intervention, family therapy and the work of R.D. Scott' was first published in the *Journal of Psychiatric and Mental Health Nursing* and is reprinted here with the kind permission of Blackwell Science Ltd.

We are grateful for the sustained support of Susan Devlin over the course of the development of this book. We hope her faith in the project has been rewarded.

Introduction to

Sean O'Brien

Sean O'Brien is one of Britain's most important poets. His most recent book of poems – *Ghost Train*, published by Oxford University Press – won the Forward Prize. He has just completed work on a new collection of poems, which will appear in 2000, published by Picador. He is the author of a controversial book of essays on contemporary poetry, entitled *The Deregulated Muse*, published by Bloodaxe, and was editor of the highly acclaimed anthology of postwar poetry, *The Firebox*. He teaches writing at Sheffield Hallam University, if the founding editor of *The Devil* magazine, and also is the poetry critic of *The Sunday Times*.

Poem for a psychiatric conference

Sean O'Brien

Thou thyself art the subject of my discourse.
Burton, preface to *The Anatomy of Melancholy*
Melancholy is . . . the character of mortality.
Burton, 'The First Partition'

i
When Marsyas the satyr played and lost
Against the god Apollo on the pipes,
The god lacked magnanimity. He skinned
The howling creature to his bones and tripes.
There in the nightmare canvas by Lorraine,
Arcadia is green, and deaf to pain.

Perhaps the melancholy are unwise
To contemplate too closely this one death,
Since they may come to think that agony's
The consequence of merely drawing breath
And that the world itself is made, to let
The mind inspect the fact it can't forget.

ii
You were staring, one teatime, into the sink
When the voice made its awful suggestion. It seems
You were really, or ought to be, somebody else
In a different house, with a different wife —
May I speak plainly? the voice enquired.
It glozed, like the serpent in Milton —
Turned out for years you'd been making it up
The kitchen, for one thing, the tiles and the draining board,

Drawing-pinned postcards and lists of to-do's,
Even the crap round the back of the freezer,
The evidence *after all spoke for itself.*
The view up the steps to the garden, for instance,
The lawn with its slow-worm, the ruinous glasshouse
Up at the top, where the hurricane left it half-standing.
The woman next door as she pinned out her washing.
The weathercock's golden irregular wink
In the breeze from the sea to its twin on the spire
A mile off. Besides, the grey channel itself
Setting out for the end of the world
Was the wrong stretch of water beside the wrong town.
You stood with your hands in your pocket and waited.
Very well, then, the God in the details disclosed:
Bus-tickets, receipts, phone numbers of people
You shouldn't have met in the pub
At the wrong time of day, the wrong year
With the wrong block of sunlight to stand
In the doorway. Your tread on the stair-carpet:
Wrong. Your skin between the freezing sheets
At dusk: an error. No matter the cause
There is error, but not correspondingly cause.

iii
The name of your case is *depression*
Although Doctor Birmingham favours
A failure of nerve. The files on the desk
In his office are fifty years old
And he, it seems, is just pretending
That he works here, sharing your gloom
And your startled gaze at the slice
Of bitter-green grass where a bottle
Keeps rolling about in the wind
At the top of the city, where everything —
Buildings, the streetmap, the people —
Has run out of steam and delivered the ground
To an evil Victorian madhouse
Complete with cupola and coalhole,
Which may or may not have shut down,
Though the bus shelter waits at the gate.

The overcooked smell is like weeping,
The cries are like nursery food
And the liverish pain on the wailing walls

Is a blatant incitement to stop being good.
Call for Nurse Bromsgrove and Sir Stafford
Wolverhampton, call Rugeley the Porter.
There are vast misunderstandings
Lurking in the syntax by the stairs.

The worst of it is, there are rooms
Not far off, waiting and book-filled
For someone like you to arrive and possess them;
A hedge at the window, and lilacs, and past them
A street that can take a whole morning
To saunter downhill past the flint walls and ginnels
Adding up to harmless privacy. This perhaps
Is what some of the mad people contemplate,
Reading their hands on a bench in the park
In their ill-fitting clothes, as if someone must come
To explain and restore and say *Put that behind you.*

1

The construction of mind and madness: from Leonardo to the Hearing Voices Network

Phil Barker

THE PROVOCATIVE SILENCE

Leonardo represents one of the most recognizable, yet least known, figures in history. The wisdom of all the ages of man emanates from his self-portrait in the Turin Royal Library. But is it really Leonardo; and, if so, what do we really know of him?

Leonardo serves as the ideal symbol of the dilemmas surrounding power and authority in psychiatry. Long after his death, figures as diverse as Vasari, Goethe, Michelet, Pater, Valery and, most significantly, Freud, claimed to know something of the un-knowable. That of which we are uncertain, we are obliged to invent. However, the drive towards 'invention' implies motivation. Turner (1993) wondered what, *exactly*, each of these 'authorities' gained from pretending to know someone whom they had never really *known*? 'Was it that each writer needed something from him?' (Turner, 1993: 3). In psychiatry, we might ask: what is the core *need* that leads to such diverse human initiatives as manipulation, control, exploitation, persecution, dismissal and disparagement, not to mention the *invention* of persons?

Perhaps his sheer ineffability makes Leonardo a useful symbol for madness. He represents the challenge of a human mystery: something that intrigues, yet at the same time generates fear – the paradox incarnate. In his notebooks Leonardo recorded 'do not reveal if liberty is precious to you'. All the evidence suggests that his resolve never wavered. So resolutely did he repel preying eyes that they fell, perforce, to elaboration, extrapolation *and* invention. His copious notes, recorded over 35 years – some in his noted mirror writing – were designed to reveal nothing of their creator: nothing of his personal feelings, daily schedules and certainly nothing of his many relationships with others. The universal man possessed a penetrating brilliance only in some areas, keeping all else in the obscurity of silence. Even the image of the ageing, tired man with the flowing beard of the prophet is, almost beyond doubt, not that of Leonardo. This is the 'too-good-to-be-true' Leonardo, the embodiment of wisdom in the shadow of extinction. This may not be the waning genius, stricken by a cerebrovascular accident, trailing silently around the Doge's Palace, but the icon that all post-Enlightenment minds *wanted* to be Leonardo.

Who will ever know for certain? Yet what we do know is that one of his biographers, Freud – the ambitious human scientist – saw fit to turn a blind eye to mistranslation and errors of historical fact, to hold his allegiance to an essentially intuitive diagnosis of Leonardo's homosexuality (Turner, 1993: 145). In that sense Freud's essay on Leonardo (1964) sets the scene for this text. We *desire* to know others, and *need* to fulfil ourselves through the explication of others. Often, however, the result is exasperation when we encounter, not an image of others, but a distorting mirror of ourselves. Does all of this lead to the 'invention of individual persons' or even the creation of a whole genus of humanity? Those with something worth concealing have long sought to conceal it. The ineffability of madness may explain how the efforts of those who sought to reveal it, have become – historically – all the more frenetic, calculating and obviously mischievous.

THE NATURE OF POWER AND AUTHORITY

Power comes in various forms – few of them are *not* disguises. The assumption that the discipline of psychiatry is a specialist area of knowledge, intrinsically confers access to some expert knowledge; and knowledge *means* power. That access appears to apply to all employed, however lowly, within this broad church. Psychiatry purports to hold the key to the riddles of human nature – even when, with hindsight, some of these insights (like Freud's on Leonardo) are dubious, if not erroneous. As a result, the knowledge base, in many circles, assumes great importance and, by implication, powers of human attorney. The relationship between psychiatry and the power of law – as in the exercise of mental health legislation – represents one such sphere of influence. How the various agents of psychiatric authority handle that body of information (not all of it worthy of the title 'knowledge') effects another strain of power. The Shavian dictum that all professionalism is a *conspiracy* against the laity, may have been stimulated by a clash with legalese and medical jargon, but is thrown into its sharpest relief in psychiatry. The control exercised over the layperson's access to psychiatric information – including, often, even the name of the particular diagnostic peephole through which the person is viewed – represents one of simplest, yet potent, power tactics. These examples of the sophisticated (as in law) and singular (as in information control) dimensions of psychiatric authority signify, perhaps, the commonest, core, characteristic of power: the ability to influence.

Historically, the power of institutional psychiatry (or more specifically, the psychiatrist) has been described as akin to that of the plantation owner: 'the power of the psychiatric bureaucrat rises with the size of the institutional system he controls and the number of patients he commands' (Szasz, 1974: 36). Although there have been numerous changes to the organization of psychiatric care, the psychiatrist's audit of available beds (fields?) remains one of the more telling indices of psychiatric power. This applies even in the case of community-based psychiatrists, who 'hold' beds as a last-stop means of dealing with difficult cases in the natural community.

Organized denial of any social responsibility for the care of people who might be deemed 'mentally disordered' has a long history. Although Antiquity had no asylums, the Greeks and Romans modelled an early version of some North American and British attitudes to 'community care'. Plato advocated that: 'if a man is mad he shall not be at large in the city, but his relations shall keep him at home in any way which they can; or if not, let them pay a penalty' (Rosen, 1968: 129).

The slow transition from stocks, to madhouse, to asylum, to hospital, over the centuries offered many opportunities to rehearse their knowledge of the ailment, and its alleviation. Psychiatrists – and before them the alienists and soul-doctors – had long nurtured ambitions to 'manage' the mentally ill (*sic*). However, by the Second World War, this image of the psychiatrist, as a utopian social engineer, had become fairly well established and, more importantly, was strongly supported.

> The gospel that men like Menninger, Lasswell and others were preaching was arrogant and grasping: they claimed that Lord Acton's famous phrase should be amended to read: Power corrupts, and absolute power corrupts absolutely – except psychiatrists. (Szasz, 1974: 216)

The wisdom of hindsight allows us to smile (at least) at some of the 'knowledge' that was once passed off as psychiatric wisdom. When Krafft-Ebbing sat down to reflect on the possible aetiology of general paralysis of the insane (GPI) in 1877, he considered 'sexual dissipation' but did not mention syphilis. More interestingly, he listed other such diverse 'causes' as: 'the menopause, trauma to the head, excessive heat and cold, fright, alcoholism, exhaustion as a result of earning a living and the *smoking of ten to twenty Virginia cigars daily*' (Rosen, 1968: 47; emphasis added). Shall we look back in another 100 years with a similar incredulity at today's medical researchers, huddled around monitors showing images of 'blood flow in schizophrenic brains', believing they were unravelling not only the mystery of the physiology of 'hearing voices', but also its human meaning.

In Szasz's view the Second World War saw the enlistment of psychiatry, regrettably emphasizing the welfare of the group over the individual. More recently, psychopharmacology and community psychiatry extended the power dimension – each of the developments carrying: 'their own moral and philosophical judgements about the nature of man and human relations' (Szasz, 1974: 217).

Community psychiatry is perceived widely as a new phenomenon, a child of the ageing father of de-institutionalization. Not only does it have slightly older roots, but may derive from a more dubious moral philosophy. The mental hygiene movement in the USA might be cited as the true source of society's desire to deal with mental disorder 'at source' – in the community. More importantly, it too derives, undoubtedly, from a more aged source. Comte, who first coined the term sociology in 1830, believed that 'the purpose of the establishment of a social philosophy is to *re-establish order* in society' (Hayek, 1955; emphasis added). The appropriate means, in Comte's view, was through attempting to explain and *control* human behaviour 'scientifically', through positivism. In Szasz's view (1974), the behaviourist engineer of Comte's day, who construed himself as a 'social physicist', 'today wears the mask of the public health physician working for the mental health of the community, the nation, the whole world' (p. 221).

THE MECHANICS OF POWER AND AUTHORITY

This crude sketch of the history of the effort to explicate and manage madness betrays something of the lineage of power and authority in psychiatry. Much of the power *dynamic* in psychiatry involves a complex of relationships. At one level it involves the power relations among the professional agents of psychiatry – between nurses, who have privileged, and direct, access to patients – and doctors, whose power over patients is often exerted only vicariously – through nurses. These two groups have long enjoyed their own 'power struggles' – rarely public, but more often covert – as in the 'doctor–nurse game' (Stein, 1967), where nurses *pretend* to 'follow' the doctor's instruction, but – through their power over the environment of care – continue to exercise their autonomy. Doctors are similarly complicit, assuming that their orders are being followed to the letter, but turning a blind eye to any, or all, interpretations.

More recently, other 'mental health workers' from the 'multi-disciplinary team' have joined these two agencies, the internal politics of health care delivery gaining a new depth. The most troublesome power dynamic, however, lies between the professional agents and the patient – and less obviously family – who rarely has any power base, despite all the urging to 'empowerment' from various 'Patients' Charters'. The complex business of *caring for* or *controlling*, far less *curing*, people in mental distress raises a huge mirror to the professional soul, reflecting much of what needs to be done to realize such lofty aims.

In her explication of the concept of 'participation' in health care, Cahill (1996) identified five 'attributes' which were essential for participation to occur:

1 A relationship needed to exist.
2 The knowledge, information or competence gap, between the practitioner and patient, needed to be narrowed.
3 Power needed to be surrendered *to a degree.*
4 Selective intellectual and/or physical activities needed to occur (which would lead to)
5 Some positive benefit accruing to the patient.

Cahill noted that these characteristics acknowledged the 'tidal' nature of most health care services, which responded to the dynamic processes of care itself, and also the shifting status of the person, influenced by numerous other factors, not least the 'severity of illness' and the person's desire to participate. Cahill noted that despite the rhetoric of empowerment and facilitation of independence in health care, the need for professionals, such as nurses, to relinquish their power (or at least some of it) was central to the achievement of 'participation'. Where this commitment to surrendering power was absent, role conflict would emerge and the patient's 'voice' would be ignored.

The idea that professionals not only might, but arguably *should*, surrender some of their power suggests the need to revise the ground rules for the relationship. Holding or surrendering power does not occur in a vacuum, and reflects key dimensions of the relationship. Without reflecting on the nature of this dynamic, and opportunities for participation, collaboration, even partnerships (Cahill, 1996), the agents of psychiatry may only be able to glimpse their charges through a glass darkly. Even within that process, however, they may gain a fleeting – but all too clear – glimpse of themselves, reflected in the human tragedies enacted before them. Such glimmerings of the reality of the power dynamic may be sufficient to deter them from exploring any further. For, as Sullivan noted: 'we are all much more simply human than otherwise, be we happy and successful, contented and detached, miserable or mentally disordered, or whatever' (Sullivan, 1953: 6). Although it does not seem difficult to empathize with the dispossessed, it is remarkable how easily professionals blind themselves to Sullivan's dictum, failing to see themselves as a reflection of the dispossessed.

Although it might appear axiomatic that 'we are more alike than different', there has long existed a contrary view that sanity and madness are antithetical experiences:

> Psychiatrists never tire of telling us that there is an unbridgeable gulf between some people and the rest of us. Karl Jaspers called it an abyss of difference. No human bond can span it. Some people are 'strange, puzzling, inconceivable, uncanny, incapable of empathy, sinister, frightening: it is impossible to approach them as equals', in Manfred Bleuler's words. Both he and Jaspers are talking about schizophrenia – over one in ten of us according to orthodox psychiatry. (Laing, 1985: 6)

Laing was renowned for his capacity to relate to the 'unrelatable'. The demise of his reputation may be the result, in part, of an almost instinctive tendency on the part of his colleagues to decry his compassion – even to the point of professional assassination. The apparent ease with which he drew the mentally dispossessed toward him, shamed all who held such people at a distance (Kotowicz, 1996). The other part of Laing's demise as an influential voice is more complex: part self-destruction and part redundancy. As the buoyant optimism of the 1960s gave way to the economies of vision which heralded the yuppiedom of the 1980s, what 'worked' – in terms of changing people – largely replaced the need to understand them.

Power issues surface in almost every area of psychiatric practice, but are most acute in areas where people have been manifestly robbed of control over their lives – or even their experience – such as victims of sexual abuse or torture. Here, the need for emphasis upon choice and some sense of control over events – although important in every area of psychiatric practice – assumes prominence. It is ironic that in an age when – at least in political terms – the importance of having and exercising a 'voice' has never been greater, those who have unconventional 'voices of conscience' – people deemed to 'suffer from auditory hallucinations' – are systematically marginalized. Or, at least institutional psychiatry tries to maintain its traditional hold over 'the voice(s)' which psychiatry has reframed as pathology. Laing's grievous sin – and Sullivan's before him – was to listen to people and their voices; expecting perhaps to learn something. More recent 'voices' in the Laingian and Sullivanian tradition – Marius Romme and Sondra Escher – gained the most unsympathetic of hearings for their text on *Accepting Voices* (1993). The reviewer from the *British Medical Journal* found much to disturb the professional mind, in the idea of 'listening' to people who 'heard voices', concluding that Romme and Escher's method of finding meaning in 'hearing voices' (auditory hallucinations) was 'dangerous' (Cochrane, 1994).

REVISITING THE PANOPTICON: WHO IS WATCHING WHOM?

The dynamics of power are – paradoxically – most evident, yet invisible, in the institutional system – or the *total* institution described by Goffman (1961). Within institutional psychiatry, the staff – or at least some of them – are as much trapped by the mechanisms of control that they enforce as the patients (*sic*) whose lives are so controlled. Goffman described how the various processes involved in detailing and monitoring the patient – which objectify the person – are designed, ultimately to monitor the staff:

> just as an article being processed through an industrial plant must be followed by a paper shadow showing what has been done and by whom, what is to be done, and who had the responsibility for it, so a *human object*, moving, say, through a mental hospital system, must be followed by a chain of informative receipts detailing what has been done to and by the patient and who had most recent responsibility for him. (Goffman, 1961: 73; emphasis added)

Although Goffman's observations are more than 40 years old, they resonate clearly with the increasingly bureaucratic system of care which is: 'rooted heavily in paranoia [and] is prevalent in any health organization today, and even more so in psychiatric units' (Fagin, 1998). Indeed, given the mounting criticisms of staff for their 'mismanagement, neglect and shoddy practices' (Fagin, 1998: 122), the requirement to 'shadow' the patient, through various paper exercises, increases, almost daily.

> Nurses, particularly, are asked to spend over half of their clinical time filling out, amongst many others, 'nursing processes', accident forms, cash withdrawal forms, special observation forms, Care Programme Approach forms, diet sheets, budget pro forma, as well as inputting questionably confidential personal data into information networks. The main purpose of all this activity is often experienced by staff as having one main objective: to prove to the inquisitor, often feared and powerful, that tasks have been completed according to pre-set standards. The fear is that if there is no written proof, no objective means of answering probing questions, responsibility will fall back on that member of staff, and their livelihood, career and peer-esteem will be threatened. (Fagin, 1998: 117)

This clinical vignette exemplifies the paradox of the Panopticon, in the later twentieth century. The staff who are employed, at the most basic level, to monitor patients (*sic*) are themselves, increasingly, the subject of monitoring. The predictions of Orwell and Huxley assume a new significance.

This reference by Fagin to nurses is interesting, if only for the fact that a psychiatrist should devote so many lines to such a lowly member of the psychiatric team. It is not unusual to read whole psychiatric texts, finding not a single reference to these 'invisible carers'. Is this something to do with most nurses – even in psychiatry – being women, and therefore lower in the authority order than their predominantly male psychiatrist colleagues (cf Colliere, 1986)? Or is it a function of the servile (womanly) status of their work, which is assumed to have no significant effect on the outcome of psychiatric care? It is notable that R.D. Laing's first study of people in psychosis,[1] involved the development of a therapeutic milieu in an aged, and impoverished Glasgow asylum (Laing *et al.*, 1955). Although the idea of creating a more convivial, socially stimulating and ordinarily 'human' environment was Laing's, those left with the 24 hour responsibility for *enacting* the facilitation of this milieu were nurses. To his credit, Laing did acknowledge the importance of their contribution. One could take the view that, from that experiment onwards, Laing gave up the practice of medicine, and devoted himself to *nursing*:[2] nourishing those in his care, rather than controlling or otherwise trying to change them.

Almost 40 years after Laing's early experiment in 'caring' for people in schizophrenia, another young Celtic psychiatrist has written about his direct experience of people in psychosis, and of his own epistemological insecurity. Regrettably, although Thomas (1997) notes – in his acknowledgements – the contribution made by two nursing colleagues 'in helping turn some of the ideas developed in this book into practice', 'nursing' and 'care' do not appear in the index. Moreover, there is virtually no further reference to either in *The Dialectics of Schizophrenia*. Thomas does, however, note in his introduction, the findings of a significant study of the 'experience' of psychiatry, by Rogers, Pilgrim and Lacey (1993). In this study of over 500 people who had at least one in-patient admission to a psychiatric hospital, *one-third* of the sample said that they had found psychiatric nurses to be 'the most helpful group'. Alternatively, only 12 per cent of the sample cited psychiatrists as 'helpful', but 21 per cent found psychiatrists 'the most unhelpful', and 38 per cent found psychiatrists' attitudes 'unhelpful or *very unhelpful*'. Such a remarkable rejection of psychiatrists, and such startling differences in the values attributed to nurses and psychiatrists, might be part of the reason why nursing and nurses is not discussed as a core part of the psychiatric canon. Foucault (1971) might well have said that the belief in the centrality of psychiatric medicine in 'helping' people in mental distress, and the core value of psychiatric medicine (to the virtual exclusion of all else), is a 'gigantic pretence'. It is all part of the 'system of exclusion' which is linked to the core system of psychiatric power; and the 'ensemble of rules' which produce and sustain it (Fernandez-Armesto, 1997).

Medicine may well be sustained by its own culture of supremacy, if not also superiority (see Fagin below). In his text, Thomas commented that, despite the reference to 'psychotherapists' in the Rogers *et al.* study, 'only a very small proportion of in-patients are likely to be under the care of a psychotherapist, whereas all in-patients will be *under the care of a psychiatrist*' (Thomas, 1997, p. 4; emphasis added). It is not mere semantics to note that all in-patients are *in the care* of nurses, whereas none are *in* the care of psychiatrists. However, all patients are *under* the psychiatrist's care, in the same way that all prisoners (in Britain) are detained *at her Majesty's pleasure*. Thomas appears to be suggesting that psychiatrists care (directly) for their patients when, patently, this can never be even the logistical truth. The psychiatrist's attitude to the service, of which he is only a part (however important) is also noted in Thomas's introduction. When he reviewed his experience of taking up a new job he talked about '*my* catchment area' and later '*my* in-patient beds'. Thomas also noted, (perhaps inadvertently) his attitude towards a young male and a young female patient, the former described as 'a young Afro-Caribbean *man*' and the latter as an 'eighteen-year-old *girl*'. In Thomas's case, these are probably no more than a careless use of the language. In general, however, the attitude of psychiatrists to *their* patients can often appear patronizing, especially in relation to gender; hence Szasz's reference to plantation owners, and the vote of low confidence from the people 'experiencing psychiatry', in the Rogers *et al.* study.

Some of these issues might well have been part of Peplau's obvious anger towards her colleagues who, by her observation, continued to publish books and papers, in which they cited medical authorities, but rarely cited their nursing colleagues' work (Peplau, 1995). Peplau, who 40 years ago developed a nursing *method* grounded in the theory of interpersonal relations (Peplau, 1952), appeared to be growing impatient with her professional colleagues. In her view, many nurses continue to function as a mere *extension* of medical practice (the 'medical-expressive role'), or wanted to model themselves ever more in the likeness of psychiatrists. A single reference to nursing theory or research in a psychiatric paper or text would be a publishing event. The citation of the work of psychiatrists is, in Peplau's view, almost *de rigeur* in the writing of nurses.[3]

It would be negligent to assume that nurses and psychiatrists are always on the same side, in terms of the power struggle in psychiatry. Psychiatrists may well exercise control over (their) patients, but rarely, if ever, do this directly. The power of the psychiatrist has always been exercised vicariously, through the ministrations of nurses. This was as true in John Connolly's day, as it is today: '. . . all his [the physician's] plans, all his care, all his personal labour, must be counteracted, if he has attendants who will not observe his rules' (Connolly, 185: 37). Consequently, nurses exercise a power which they do not, actually, own. In the process, described by Goffman, they may be disempowered – being left at the 'care-face', to deal with all the human distress associated with madness, whether emanating from the patient, or friends and family; and being required also to deal with the various critical demands of practice coming from management. Nurses, in Peplau's view, have always been the more important agencies for 'growth and development', but have also been seen as marginal to the core business of psychiatry. During a recorded conversation, I asked her to tell me about her early career, when she 'worked with Harry Stack Sullivan at Chestnut Lodge'. Peplau replied, 'Why . . . I never *worked* with Sullivan . . . I *worked* at Chestnut Lodge (as a trainee analyst) but not *with* Sullivan. I mean, I was a nurse *and* a woman. He wouldn't have me in the room!'

Although much has changed in the 50 years since Peplau's experience of Sullivan, it is relatively easy to take the view that the attitudinal gap between psychiatrists and the nurses they rely upon to *do* their bidding, has not. It may not be the case that young psychiatrists like Thomas have a disdain for nurses – indeed I believe quite the opposite is true. However, he would be unlikely to even think about discussing 'nursing' and 'caring', since these two activities – and the philosophies that underpin them – have no historical location in the psychiatric canon.[4] Despite the countless acres of paper which annually are produced, upon which are documented the psychiatrists 'relationship with patients', the everyday fact is that such relationships are fleeting. Indeed, they may not even be relationships, but might be defined, more appropriately, as 'interactions' – designed, for example, to elicit answers to a mental status examination. A patient noted sagely: 'when he [the doctor] asks me "how I am", I know he isn't interested in *me*, as such. He simply wants to know if the drugs he gave me last time are working.'

THE CONTENT OF PSYCHIATRY: THE MENU OF POWER AND AUTHORITY

Yet, despite the fleeting nature of psychiatrists' relations with patients,[5,6] the layperson probably still believes that psychiatric patients receive psychoanalysis, or have their minds explored in depth, and at length, by a sage and kindly soul-doctor. From where did this cultural fiction originate? Cinema, television and the popular press have all played their part. The long-running BBC radio programme *In the Psychiatrist's Chair* features the Irish psychiatrist Anthony Clare in intimate – and often disarmingly intrusive exploration – of the *psyches* and childhood experiences of notable, public figures. Although Clare's radio persona has promoted an image of himself as an advocate of psychoanalysis, his professional writing betrays a rejection of the value of psychodynamic therapy and, especially, psychoanalysis (Clare, 1976). Even if it is correct to assume that most psychiatrists now spend little time with their patients, and are largely intent on determining which drugs to prescribe, this might be an unpalatable truth for a society which has invested so much importance in the soul-doctor. More importantly, such a truth might severely damage the reputation of a discipline whose representatives comment regularly in the popular press on all manner of human foibles, failings and fatalities: from love, sexuality and relationships, to cults, crime and dying. Of course, there are notable authorities in each of these fields who *are* psychiatrists. However, the cultural illusion is that these areas are the province of *all* psychiatrists. Perhaps, society needs psychiatrists to have such authority, as much as psychiatrists wish to perpetuate Foucault's 'gigantic pretence'.

Nurses, on the other hand, are often depicted as the least powerful of the mental health professionals, and are probably the last people who would be sought to offer a public comment on the social context of mental distress, far less sex, drugs, relationships and life in general. Nurses are the 'footsoldiers' in the fight against madness. Theirs is not to reason why, far less comment. However, it would be grossly incorrect to say that, just because no power is attributed to nurses, they do not own power, by dint of their position within the psychiatric church.

Nurses possess the power to manage the life-space (or milieu) of patients in hospital and, increasingly – through supervision registers – that of patients in the community. Their social status is commonly dismissed as menial – one notch above the untrained staff (or nursing aides) who spend a lot of time caring for patients, and two notches above the cleaners, who devote a lot of effort to maintaining the patients' environment (at least in hospital). There is a popular view, however, that nurses *only* engage in these forms of management out of fear, or as defensive practices. Some, like Fagin – a senior British psychiatrist – perceive nurses as almost helpless – perhaps even 'cannon fodder' for the psychiatric war against mental illness:

> Nurses are often at the forefront of any hospital reorganization, but are not usually the instigators. They have direct contact with the patient, more so than any other mental health professional, and yet they are the working class of the psychiatric social structure, and have to respond to edicts from their superiors without much say or influence. Many have likened nursing to the military professions. Adherence to rules and deference to *superiors* are deeply entrenched in the nursing psyche. (Fagin, 1998: 118–19; emphasis added).

In the days of the large, socially isolated, asylum, there existed a *patriarchal* psychiatrist who, traditionally, would 'run' the old asylum; taking an interest in the affairs of staff and patients, all of whom were part of his (invariably) small empire. Some of these figures were revered, others despised. In most cases, the relationship between the 'physician superintendent' and the staff was 'master–servant'. Whether nurses chose, or were required, to be deferential, and the extent to which anything has changed, with the move to 'community mental health teams' (CMHTs), is a matter of dispute.

In a recent study of such mental health teams, Morall (1998) showed that the power (if not class) differential between psychiatrists and nurses has hardly shifted, and the primacy of the psychiatrist – and now the psychologist – remained. In Morall's study four of the five consultant psychiatrists and all the psychologists, indicated that they considered this (diagnosis) to be the fundamental element in the demarcation between senior and junior groups of occupations in the CMHT. A new power struggle appears to be developing between psychologists and nurses. A psychologist voiced:

> her concern about the capabilities of CPNs to deliver such specialist treatments as, for example, cognitive therapy. The CPNs need to be supervised, she suggests, to stop them doing 'cracker things' and to prevent her own discipline from being held in disrepute. Furthermore, she recommends that the role of the CPN should be confined to one of providing 'support'. (Morall, 1998: 103)

In Morall's study the impatience voiced more than a century ago by John Connolly, has passed through the hands of his medical descendants, to clinical psychologists. Bean and Mounser (1989) suggested that the move of psychiatry to the community would, ultimately, extend the empire of psychiatric medicine, since by broadening the scope and membership of the community mental health team: 'these auxiliary staff (social workers, nurses, psychologists, behavioural therapists and occupational therapists) now emulate the medical approach and, in so doing, reinforce the credibility of the power of psychiatry' (Bean and Mounser, 1989: 168).

These developments illustrate some of the internal politics of the 'mental health team', and betray the jockeying for status, and power over patients, which continues unabated. Fagin's observation was interesting for the distinction he made (implicitly) between 'superiors' and 'seniors'. The 'superiority' of those who issue 'edicts' is predicated more on their power than any other quality. Regrettably, despite the implicit 'power' of nurses, within the 'doctor–nurse game', there has been little in the way of opposition, from nurses, to the growing demands for nurses – in all Westernized countries – to assume more power over patients. The 'voice' of psychiatric nursing appears now to differ little from the ventriloquial voice of the psychiatrist.

Traditionally, those who have most often issued edicts to nurses – or spoken *for* them – have been doctors. Part of Fagin's concern for nurses involves the manner by which the psychiatrist's power to orchestrate the institution – and instigate reorganization – has begun to be transferred, as a function of managerialism: 'More and more of the planning activities were passed on to a succession of managers rather than clinicians, often more conscious of financial rather than clinical considerations' (1998: 114).

Fagin may well be speaking for many clinicians[7] in psychiatry, who fear that their power – and autonomy – has been irreparably eroded by the import of the business ethic into health care, along with the rich, but arguably empty, rhetoric of 'managerialism'.

Here may lie the final, ironic, irony: that the power and authority which psychiatric medicine, and the soul-doctors before that, has long prized, may have been 'prised' from its grasp by a retinue of grey suits.

LEONARDO BIDS DESCARTES FAREWELL

Through what appears, to today's mind, a fairly simple contrivance, Descartes created the modern concept of the mind, as distinct from the body. In Wilber's (1997) view Descartes may be one of the few representatives of 'Western Vedanta' who developed an intellectual awareness that was highly focused on its own source, 'i.e. witnessing subjectivity, the pure self' (Wilber, 1997: 308). Such 'philosophical inquiry opens onto contemplative awareness: the mind itself subsides in the vast expanse of primordial awareness, and the philosophia gives way to contemplatio' (Wilber, 1997: 309).

Such 'philosophical inquiry' was, however, to be the 'modern' project – which has grown into contemporary efforts to equate the 'mind' with the neurochemical activity of the brain. The ideas, which people today (and especially tomorrow) hold about 'the mind' will be influenced, to varying degrees, by contemporary neuroscience and psychology. When Descartes made his original assertion over 300 years ago, his philosophy (ultimately) effected a 'change of mind' about the mind within society. Which thought returns us to Leonardo and his most (in)famous biographer. It has largely been overlooked that Freud did not acknowledge that he was a 'late-modern' mind, looking through the mists of time for his reflection in the Renaissance mind of Leonardo. Indeed, apart from the obvious fact that the intervening 400 years must make for almost impossible comparisons, it seemed never to have occurred to Freud, that Leonardo might not even have possessed anything akin to the 'mind', which Descartes' modernist project had begun to create. Turner (1993) noted that 'Freud . . . was wont to generalize from specific clinical cases, and in a brilliant essay proposed that on the assumption that a Viennese mind in 1900 must approximate a Florentine mind of circa 1500, Leonardo was fit to be a dead analysand' (p. 132). Freud's brilliant essay reminds one of the Irish saying 'facts should never get in the way of a good story'. Indeed, the history of the psychiatric drive towards the imperial control of madness, if not all everyday life, suggests that many a blind eye has been turned to fact, and many a rule reframed to allow the continued exploration and domination of the interior. Increasingly, however, people who have been long-term recipients of psychiatric services – many describing themselves as 'survivors' of the psychiatric machine – are taking back the personal power which, first, madness and then, psychiatry took from them. One such group is the international Hearing Voices Network. One of its members drew attention to the weak standing of psychiatry as an agent of 'treatment for mental illness'. His voice – which is finding echoes all around the globe – serves as the best conclusion to this, first, introduction to the text. Speaking of the concept of mental *illness* Coleman argued:

> The World Health Organization have clearly stated that in order to classify an illness there must be what are known as the three commonalties. These are the commonality of cause, the commonality of progression and the commonality of outcome. It is abundantly clear that within so-called mental illness that none of these commonalties occur. The cause of mental illness is still fiercely contested, even amongst those who believe in a biological construction there is much controversy between those who argue the chemical cause, those who believe in a genetic causation and those who assume that it is a physical brain disorder. (Coleman, 1998: 18)

In Coleman's view, people whose experiences require to be understood, instead, are defined, classified and ultimately stripped of (at least) some of their humanity, through being 'psychiatrized' (in Morall's terms). He recognizes that if people like himself are to recover their personal power, then that power must be taken back: 'if sanity is in the eye of the beholder then we must make sure that the establishment is no longer the beholder' (Coleman, 1998).

A mature 'mind' might be content to look back on Leonardo and simply gasp in astonishment, rather than fumble with some pretence at knowledge of the man. Coleman may, or may not, know himself (and his mind) better than anyone else. What seems clear, is that he – like Leonardo – has resisted, and looks set to continue to do so, attempts by others to gain entry to his private world, or at least without his permission. The door into the private world of madness may not even be ajar, far less open. That may explain psychiatry's traditional tendency to try to break it down.

NOTES

1 I appreciate that people are more likely to be 'in' this state, from time to time, rather than 'have' it – somehow as part of their identity or 'self'.
2 In most dictionaries the term nursing is recognized to be a derivative of 'nourish' (nurish) – where someone is brought up under certain conditions designed to 'foster, tend or cherish (a thing)' promoting its growth and development (*Shorter Oxford English Dictionary*, 1962).
3 As a psychiatric nurse, my view is, clearly, a partial one. A casual perusal of the two literatures should, however, redeem me from any accusation of gross partiality.
4 This is, of course, part of the reason why Laing appeared to break the psychiatric code.
5 Over 20 years ago the British psychiatrist Albert Kushlick described psychiatrists (and psychologists) as 'hit and runners', or DC10s: they give 'direct care to the patient for about ten minutes, then fly off somewhere else'.
6 Recent economic studies conducted in the USA show that psychiatrists, once strongly associated with the practice of psychotherapy, have all but been driven out of this role by the power of the health insurance companies, who regard them as too expensive. 'Psychiatrists now largely spend their time doing mental exams and prescribing drugs, having apologised to their physician brothers for ever having left the fold of medicine' (Berg, 1998).
7 The term 'clinician' could be applied to any clinical practitioner, but in managerial language this is, usually, understood as meaning the psychiatrist.

REFERENCES

Bean, P. and Mounser, P. (1989) Community care and the discharge of patients from mental hospitals. *Law Med Health Care*, **17**(2): 166–73.
Berg, L. (1998) The Economics of Psychotherapy. Paper presented at the conference 'The Future of Psychotherapy 2000', at Esholt Hall, Yorkshire.
Cahill, J. (1996) Patient participation: a concept analysis. *Journal of Advanced Nursing*, **24**: 561–571.
Clare, A. (1976) *Psychiatry in Dissent: controversial issues in thought and practice*. London: Tavistock Publications.
Cochrane, R. (1994) Accepting voices – a review. *British Medical Journal*, 308: 1649.
Coleman, R. (1998) *Politics of the Madhouse*. Runcorn: Handsell Publishing.
Colliere, F. (1986) Invisible care and invisible women as health care providers. *International Journal of Nursing Studies*, **23**(2): 95–112.
Connolly, J. (1856) *The Treatment of the Insane without Mechanical Restraint*. London: Smith, Elder and Co.
Fagin, L. (1998) Paranoia in institutional life: the death throes of the asylum. In H.H. Berke, S. Pierides, A. Sabbadini and S. Schneider (eds), *Even Paranoids Have Enemies: New perspectives on paranoia and persecution*. London: Routledge.
Fernandez-Armesto, F. (1997) *Truth: A History*. London: Bantam Press.
Foucault, M. (1971) *L'Ordre de discours*. Paris: Gallimard.

Freud, S. (1964) Leonardo Da Vinci and a Memory of His Childhood. From Five Lectures on Psychoanalysis, Leonardo and Other Works. In J. Strachey, A. Strachey and A. Tyson (eds), *The Standard Edition of the Complete Psychological Works of Sigmund Freud*, vol. XI. London: Hogarth Press.

Goffman, E. (1961) *Asylums: Essays on the Social Situations of Mental Patients and Other Inmates*. New York: Doubleday.

Hayek, F.A. von (1955) *The Counter-Revolution of Science: Studies on the Abuse of Reason*. Glencoe, IL: Free Press.

Kotowicz, Z. (1997) *R. D. Laing and the Paths of Antipsychiatry*. London: Routledge.

Laing, R.D., Cameron, J.L. and McGhie, A. (1955) Patient and nurse effects of environmental changes in the care of chronic schizophrenics. *Lancet*, **ii**, 1384–1386.

Laing, R. D. (1985) *Wisdom, Madness and Folly: The Making of a Psychiatrist*. London: Macmillan.

Morall, P (1998) *Mental Health and Social Control*. Whurr: London.

Peplau, H.E. (1952) *Interpersonal Relations in Nursing*. Putnam: New York.

Peplau, H.E. (1995) Another look at schizophrenia from a nursing standpoint. In: C.A. Anderson (ed.), *Psychiatric Nursing 1974–1994: the State of the Art*. St Louis: Mosby.

Rogers, A., Pilgrim, D. and Lacey, R. (1993) *Experiencing Psychiatry: Users' Views of Services*. London: MIND/Macmillan.

Romme, M. and Escher, S. (1993) *Accepting Voices*. London: MIND/Macmillan.

Rosen, G. (1968) *Madness in Society: Chapters in the Historical Sociology of Mental Illness*. London: The University of Chicago Press.

Stein, L.I. (1967) The doctor–nurse game. *Archives of General Psychiatry*, **16**: 699–700.

Sullivan, H.S. (1953) *The Conceptions of Modern Psychiatry*. New York: Norton.

Szasz, T.S. (1974) *Ideology and Insanity*. Harmondsworth: Penguin.

Thomas, P. (1997) *The Dialectics of Schizophrenia*. London: Free Association Books.

Turner, A.R. (1993) *Inventing Leonardo: The Anatomy of a Legend*. New York: Alfred A Knopf.

2

Living within and without psychiatric language games

Chris Stevenson

INTRODUCTION: THE IMPORTANCE OF LANGUAGE

> 'The time has come,' the Walrus said,
> 'To talk of many things:
> Of shoes – and ships – and sealing wax –
> Of cabbages – and kings –
> And why the sea is boiling hot –
> And whether pigs have wings.'

> ('The Walrus and the Carpenter' from
> *Through the Looking Glass* by Lewis Carroll)

During my academic career, I have become increasingly enchanted by the nature of language. I am speaking from within the post-modern turn as I write this chapter. Post-modernism is notoriously undefined and indefinable (Stevenson and Reed, 1996). I take the view that post-modernism arises as the modern takes up self-reflexivity, deconstructing 'taken for granted' ways of making sense of the world, such as grand theories, in favour of local and specific accounts; expressing reservations about foundationalism, and the acceptance of singular truths; celebrating complexity and ambiguity, inconsistencies, paradoxes and contradictions; doubting progress as a linear process. I am aware that there are alternative stories that can be told about language. I do not wish to make a truth claim here about what the best account of language consists in. Truth is problematic and not necessarily accessible through a process of scientific exploration or logical reasoning, at least from where I am standing as I write this piece. What I write is my fiction.

From the representationalist viewpoint, words are often taken to represent some external reality. Words are value-free labels that are applied to objects. The neutrality of language is assumed in professional spheres as it is seen as 'a transparent medium of scientific communication' (Crawford *et al.*, 1995: 1141). Mary Boyle, in her chapter in this book, makes a similar point in relation to the claimed neutrality of psychiatric diagnosis. 'Special words' allow professionals a way of talking about their world of practice. It is a convenient shorthand to describe a person as 'schizophrenic' or 'borderline'; to identify 'trouble at the synapse' as the cause of mental illness. Jenner, in Chapter 9, argues that diagnostic categories are meaningful in so far as they allow differentiation of things and allow intellectual content. But implicit in professional language is a notion of 'us and them'. 'On the far side of a boundary we locate individuals in psychosis, people who engage in improper talk about the world. On this side of the boundary are we, the sane, the inheritors of a shared reality' (Birch, 1996: 286). Most importantly, there is nothing inherent in the identification of difference that means that power should be given to one camp or the other. In practice, however, it lies with diagnosing professionals.

But perhaps borders are fuzzier than we routinely think. Birch (1996) points out that between England and Scotland there is a belt of debatable lands which makes the border drawn on the map only a useful fiction which exists because enough people are prepared to live with it. But once people behave as if something is the only reality, there is less opportunity to put another gloss on history. My daughter likes to stand with one foot in England and another in Scotland. She never questions whether the imaginary line on the map is accurate or helpful. Similarly, 'Pathologizing discourse does not invite us to discuss or question how a professional hegemony comes to be describing troubled individuals using the language of defect' (Birch, 1996: 287–8).

Birch (1996) argues that a single 'take' on troubled people creates negative equity for those persons, and also for the professionals with whom they interlocute. On the one hand there is the stigma of diagnosis as a catalogue of defects, on the other the therapist is stunted in her/his ability to work creatively by the limiting grammar. Balint (1957) noted that medical doctors have an apostolic function – in coaching them how to experience their illness (Birch, 1991). Such tutelage is necessarily proscribed if one story prevails. For example, the predominance of the search for a magic bullet (cure) for schizophrenia precludes the provision of information about how to construct a therapeutic interview with someone in such distress. Perhaps this indicates that it is time for another story . . .

WHY IS LANGUAGE IMPORTANT? PSYCHIATRIC GRAMMAR CONSTRUCTS THE PATIENT

Let us begin with the biological symptoms of psychiatric distress. In this we can keep company with the traditionally acknowledged 'great and good' of psychiatry. Bleuler (1911: 150) regarded auditory hallucinations as important symptoms, and observed: 'Where . . . auditory hallucinations continually dominate the clinical picture, one can practically always conclude that one is dealing with schizophrenia.' However, Bleuler's 'criteria did not lead to categorical diagnoses, as do signs and symptoms in medicine' (Jenner *et al.*, 1993: 29). Boyle (see Chapter 5) points out that psychiatric diagnosis does not follow the process of medical diagnosis. The latter relies on previous research that has identified a patterning of physical pathology and complaints which allows the inference of a disease concept, e.g., diabetes. In psychiatric diagnosis, the diagnostic labels are *followed* by a search for a pattern of diagnostic criteria. But such a search should be unnecessary as the diagnostic label's validity could only have been established in the first place if there were adequate diagnostic criteria already. Despite this problematic circularity, Schneider (1959) attempted to find clear signs and symptoms of schizophrenia, the first and second rank symptoms that are familiar to most psychiatric professionals. The quest for a science of diagnosis is well outlined by Foucault:

> In the form of the clinic, in the technique of medical examination, the disseminated power of the gaze permitted the constitution of a knowledge ability about disease, observable in symptoms and signs. The symptoms 'allow the invariable form of the disease . . . visible and invisible, to *show through*'. . . . . .Whereas a symptom *is*, a sign *says*. (1976: 92–3)

Yet biological symptoms are refracted through the prism of language, as the person *reports* their symptoms, as the professional observes and *records* symptoms, as the professional network *relays* a description of the symptoms, as the psychiatric professionals *respond* to symptoms. 'Human beings live "in language" in the same way that fish live in water' (Anderson and Goolishian, 1988: 56). 'When people describe symptoms, these descriptions are freighted with other meanings; they are a way of communicating a good deal of other business' (Crawford *et al.*, 1995: 1143). These authors go on to claim that patient records are created biographies which are fictitious, but are powerful linguistic entrapments which serve to depersonalize and disempower the patient.

There is never a 'view from nowhere' (Nagel, cited in Bruner, 1990: 14). Webb (1992: 748) cites Britton's position that 'word labels represent a classification system based on our ways of thinking about the objects concerned'. Implicit within psychiatric naming systems is a grammar in the Wittgensteinian sense. Wittgenstein (1953) defined grammar as the rules which allow us to 'engage in patterns of conjoint action' (Cronen and Lang, 1994: 18). The rules constitute a 'language game' (Wittgenstein, 1953) which can be of different kinds. In a fixed rule language game:

> an observer can detect the rules of the game through watching it being played. The rules are reconstituted by the playing of the game. Chess is a good example of a fixed rule language game. Cultural practices such as the judicial system, for example, have 'fixed rule language games'. (Stevenson and Beech, 1998: 791)

Harré (1998) has described how a grammar can constrain the possibility for reasoning and for social functioning. For example, Stevenson and Beech (1998) have described how ethical committee members were limited by the grammar of science, to an extent that they could not break away from thinking about validity and reliability in relation to a qualitative research proposal, which demanded a different form of evaluation. The committee only agreed to C.S.'s research on the grounds that it could not do any harm. Within psychiatry, there are well-rehearsed stories about what constitutes madness, the fable of the *Diagnostic and Statistical Manual*, in its latest manifestation (American Psychiatric Association, 1994); the guidance within the Mental Health Act (1983). The grammar of these particular language games consists of rules about how biological disturbance manifests itself, about the relationship (or lack of it) of madness and responsibility, about how to manage risk and dangerousness. The grammar invites certain questions of the order: 'How are you feeling today?'; 'What is the problem that brought you to the clinic?'; 'Have you thought about taking your own life?'. The psychiatric patient is constructed as sick, helpless, irresponsible, unpredictable and needy (of professional intervention). Scott (1995: 6) comments:

> in psychiatric practice [where] we are almost exclusively drawn to the negative, to what is wrong and commonly fail to realise the primary importance of positive feeling, This is an imprint of the closed attitude. It runs through psychiatry.

In a later chapter, Coleman (see Chapter 4) argues that 'the schizophrenic' is characterized as either an axe-wielding madman or a social inadequate. Stevenson and Beech (1998) give an example of an encounter between psychiatric patient and professional during which the patient makes a reality claim that extra-terrestrial forces are controlling him. The professional, who follows the language game of her/his profession, eschews a discussion of delusional material for fear it may reinforce the illness. Stalemate ensues, usually broken by the administration of medication to impose the professional's privileged view of reality on the patient. As Szasz argues later in this book (see Chapter 3), 'From the insider's point of view, state sanctioned violence is, by definition, just' (p. 43). Boyle (see Chapter 5) points out that diagnosis seems to invite certain interventions and make other actions, e.g., in the educational and spiritual domain, less likely. Szasz also states that 'The psychiatrist's power over that patient negates the possibility of a human encounter between them.' The position outlined here accords with that of Crawford *et al.* (1995) that while language is a communication tool it may also serve to confirm the power that professionals wield in relation to those who seek their help. The technical language of health care is exclusive and excluding. For example, 'to reconceptualize a reluctance to go shopping on one's own as "agoraphobia" is to perform a shift in topic which is potentially empowering for the therapist' (Crawford *et al.*, 1995: 1142). In Chapter 3, Szasz argues that the psychiatrist must view the person experiencing problems of living as a patient suffering from a serious disease in order to maintain her/his state sanctioned position.

Another way to think of this constructive process is with reference to the body-without-organs (BWO). This idea derives from the writings of some post-structural scholars, e.g., Deleuze and Guattari (1984, 1988). The BWO is a political, and not an anatomical or physiological surface upon which are inscribed discourses, defined as dialogical process, which lead to a conversational reality. For example, psychiatric medicine may inscribe the body with a discourse (of professional knowledge) of bio-pathology; of inevitable social decline; of intractability. The BWO is *territorialized* by these discourses of knowledge. Birch (1991) points out that such discourses lead to self-sustaining disabling cycles: a cycle of disqualification, where 'sufferers' and families lose their sense of expertise and defer to the opinion of psychiatric experts; a cycle of victimhood, where 'sufferers' see little hope for a socially fulfilling life; a cycle of fatalism in which the 'sufferer' and her/his social network wait for the next relapse.

In an emergent rules language game, the participants' 'ideas about how to create meanings, put words, sentences, gestures, emotions and patterns of behaviour together, arise through the playing of the game' (Stevenson and Beech, 1998: 791). For example, when children play they often make the rules up as they go along on the basis of a consensual view of what is fair. They may decide that an existing rule that a ball has to be caught cleanly can be adapted when they notice a younger child struggle. A no-bounce rule is superseded by a rule that allows the ball to bounce once before the younger child catches it (Stevenson and Beech, 1998). Within emergent rule language games, we create rules for living in coordination with others, thereby knowing how to act in given situations (Hannah, 1994). Emergent rule language games are rarely played in psychiatry.

Such a situation would allow possibilities that would undermine the power position of the psychiatric establishment. Playfully, these can be presented as Zen Koans: 'Contemplate the therapist-less client' (Birch, 1995: 224); Contemplate the patientless nurse; Contemplate the atypical schizophrenic; Contemplate the bedless psychiatrist.

When two fixed rule language games collide they often clash. There is not an existing shared grammar that can be brought into play. In these circumstances, each camp is likely to indulge itself with good guy/bad guy discourse (Birch, 1995). The two sides present their self-justificatory monologues. Seikkula (1995) points out that monologues entail a position that one thing is more right than another is. There are many examples of clashing discourses in psychiatry, but the growth in the 1950s and 1960s of alternative (not anti) psychiatry is worth visiting in some detail. Gregory Bateson was developing his communicational theory of schizophrenia (Bateson *et al.*, 1956) at a time when the 'discovery' of phenothiazines was emptying the asylums. Speaking from within psychiatric medicine, Ronnie Laing was questioning the value of existing clinical language:

> As a psychiatrist I run into a major difficulty at the outset: how can I go straight to the patients if the psychiatric words at my disposal keep the patient at a distance from me? How can one demonstrate the general human relevance and significance of the patient's condition if the words one has to use are specifically designed to circumscribe the meaning of the patient's life to a particular clinical entity? (Laing, 1960: 18)

But the most sustained battle has been between the psychiatric establishment and Thomas Szasz. As Horowitz (1996: 24) puts it, 'If there is another living psychiatrist who has suffered more professional obliquity while sustaining great public recognition, this person escapes my recognition.' In a series of papers and books published over four decades, Professor Szasz has challenged the ideas that madness is synonymous with irresponsibility; that psychiatric care is compassionate; that mental illness is other than a myth; that psychiatric 'care' should be other than by consent.

WHY DO SUCH BATTLES OCCUR?

> The prejudice of crystalline purity can only be got rid of by turning our whole point of observation. (Wittgenstein, 1953: ¶108)

Within fixed rule language games, there is an assumption that words have a function of representing an external world out there; that there is a reality that can be unproblematically captured. Words then take on a life of their own as demonstrated in a World Health Organization position statement: 'Why is the concept of schizophrenia necessary at all? Firstly, because we have the term' (World Health Organization, quoted in Szasz, 1993: 21).

Such views have been challenged by writers within the post-modern turn, who have frequently drawn on the later work of Wittgenstein (1953). Wittgenstein notes that we can choose to use words as representations, but this is a matter of preference not truth. 'When *I* use a word,' Humpty Dumpty said, in rather a scornful tone, 'it means just what I choose it to mean – neither more nor less' (*Through the Looking Glass*, Lewis Carroll). There is always a gap between the signifier and the signified. Meaning is, inevitably, deferred (Derrida, 1978). When we begin to describe a concept there is a slippage of meaning. For example, when I describe a chair it is not possible to represent the reality but only to refer to other signifiers of chairness.

> While trying to represent the real, the meaning that one is trying to communicate slips from one's grasp. We are left not with the reality, but with an approximation which, however much we try to make it 'more real', is always already deferred and irrecoverable. (Fox, 1993: 8)

Because of slippage in meaning, no text (text is not just written words but includes conversation, art, non-verbal communication etc.) has a single incontestable reading. For example, an English cricket radio commentator once famously declared, 'The batsman's Holding, the bowler's Willey'. There are telling ambiguities in psychiatric language which demonstrate the metaphorical nature of language, as well as a power dynamic: Patient means a person under treatment *and* undemanding, able to wait; Client has synonyms of ward, delinquent, dependent, orphan and minor. Szasz (1996) considers the problems of translation in relation to the work of Bleuler (1911), and concludes that the treachery of translation leads to a concept 'thought disorder'. But thought disorder can be convincingly redrawn as self conversation, likely to be characterized as disordered only with the catalyst of the psychiatrist's assessment of faulty speech. Birch (personal communication) puts this across well when he says that the language game of hallucinations cannot be played solo. I return to this issue later when considering monologue and dialogue.

A story of native American peoples (Lopez, 1986) presented by Stewart *et al.* (1991) is an example of how ideological and linguistic impasse can be overcome, how power relationships between opposing camps can be enacted differently. Lopez gathered information from the Nannamuit about wolverines, their biology and ecology, which he sent to a friend who was living with the Cree. The Cree were asked their opinions of the

Nannamuit observations. The Cree accepted the observations as accurate, whilst acknowledging that they themselves saw things differently. As Lopez relates it, his friend reminded him, 'You know how . . . they are. They said, "It could be."' Lopez summarizes (1986: 66):

> Whenever I think of this courtesy on the part of the Cree, I think of the dignity that is ours when we cease to demand the truth, and realize that the best we can have of those substantial truths that guide our lives is metaphorical – a story. And the most of it we are likely to discern comes only when we accord to one another the respect the Cree showed the Nannamuit. Beyond this – that truth reveals itself not in dogma but in the paradox, irony, and contradictions that distinguish compelling narratives – beyond this there are only failures in imagination: reductionism in science; fundamentalism in religion; fascism in politics . . .

. . .diagnosis and coercion in psychiatry? The Cree were not prepared, as the Irish saying goes, to let the facts get in the way of a good story. But what is a good story? Cronen and Lang (1994) have suggested that a story, which is coherent, which 'fits' for the parties involved, allows them to conjointly go with their lives.

RECLAIMING THE PSYCHIATRIC BODY WITHOUT ORGANS THROUGH ALTERNATIVE STORYING

If people believe that language is representational, alternative versions of events seem alien:

> Twas brillig, and the slithy toves
> Did gyre and gimble in the wabe
> All mimsy were the borogoves
> And the mome raths outgabe.
>
>   'It seems very pretty,' [Alice] said . . . 'but it's rather hard to understand!' . . . 'Somehow it seems to fill my head with ideas – only I don't exactly know what they are . . .' (*Through the Looking Glass*, Lewis Carroll)

Alice cannot understand the poem because to understand requires her to step outside existing shared language. Cronen and Lang (1994) suggest that people's grammatical abilities are informed by multiple stories which we learn to tell as part of our socialization into particular groups – the family, the profession etc. Such stories are not to be reified as truths. For Cronen and Lang (1994) one story is not naturally more powerful than another is, although we behave *as if* some stories have a stronger truth claim. In Western societies, medicine has colonized health and established a hegemony through drawing on a knowledge base that is seen as legitimate through its claim to be scientific. In relation to bio-medicine,

Foucault (1976) notes that the knowledge held by doctors about the human body, health and illness, supplies the substance by which medical dominance is established and maintained. The BWO is territorialized by such professional discourses of knowledge. Szasz, in this book, identifies that influence over others is gained through the perception that the professional has power in relation to their ability to satisfy a need. On this basis, the professional can 'influence' the patient.

Yet:

> There is no such thing as absolute power. If we can uncover the conditions that allowed a certain archaeology of knowledge to emerge we can more easily reject knowledges as *necessary* accounts without rejecting them as *possible* accounts. Once knowledges are exposed as discourses, ways of talking about our lives, alternative discourses might more easily come into play. (Stevenson and Beech, 1998: 795)

For example, Gould (1981) has debunked the foundations of science through a historical exploration of research findings. Whilst accepted in their time, the research conclusions have turned out to be driven by the desire to identify people as inferior to white Anglo-Saxons in respect of their criminality and intelligence. In this book, Suman Fernando tracks the history of racial differential in psychiatry. He argues that there is a confounding of myth (big, black and dangerous), rooted in imperialism, and fact (psychiatric presentation) in determining diagnosis (usually schizophrenia) and treatment plans (frequently compulsory detention and seclusion) for people from black populations.

The surface of the BWO, where inscription takes place, is also the place where resistance occurs. It can be de-territorialized, enabling it to become something other than that which it was as a consequence of its original inscription. How? Crawford *et al.* (1995: 1143) state that:

> Clinical practice is the intersection where meanings of the world converge. The health worker (theories), the client (stories and narratives) and culture (myths, rituals and themes) all converge in the linguistic interaction. Acknowledging this enables the health care worker not to pathologize or psychologize problems that might better be conceptualized in political or social terms.

The psychiatric BWO can be inscribed by discourses of academics, clinicians, friends, parents, lovers, colleagues, the media etc. Such inscriptions can be powerful or powerless, invoke negative or positive images of those within psychiatric systems. For example, Deleuze (1969) has a different discourse of schizophrenia that goes beyond an illness description to note that schizophrenia is a possibility for thought. In the wider societal context, 'media schizophrenia' (Birch, 1991) inscribes people with schizophrenia as 'wasted lives' in which the sufferer is condemned to be controlled by drug therapy. Johnstone (1994) has pointed out that the prevalent view presented by the media is of the mentally ill as dangerous, unpredictable and irresponsible. There is an active lay language of madness – a lexicon of lunacy that has stretched through the centuries (Szasz, 1993). Ron Coleman in Chapter 4 provides an evocative insider view of psychiatric illness, responsibility and power. In his articulate presentation and productivity he threatens the usual inscription on the psychiatric BWO of attributes such as lack of motivation, irresponsibility, ignorance etc.

PROFESSIONAL POSITIONING

Shotter (1998) takes the view that language and action are inseparable. We act into situations and it is only then that we try to make sense *of* the situation: 'in the beginning was the deed' (Wittgenstein, 1980: 31). Professionals have (largely) ignored their 'embodied embeddedness' (Shotter, 1998: 34), because they have been subject to their particular disciplinary gaze.

> A discipline '. . .produces subjected and practised, "docile" bodies' (Foucault, 1979, p. 138), bodies which have lost the ability to question their own praxis. Beguiled by the tendency of our disciplinary discourses to 'form the objects of which they speak' (Foucault, 1972, p. 49), we find it difficult to find our own, spontaneous academic talk problematic. (Shotter, 1998: 37)

Thus, it is non-standard psychiatric practice to reflect on the process by which the practitioner, or discipline, has arrived at a particular position. One exception is Reed (1996: 255) who suggests that:

> The assumptions, knowledge claims and practices which are prevalent within the fields of psychiatry and psychotherapy have emerged from within particular historical, cultural and political contexts, and claims to universality should be regarded with scepticism. Feminist commentators have drawn attention to the patriarchal assumptions reflected in much psychological and psychotherapeutic theory (Perelberg and Miller, 1990) . . .

Another is Jenner (see Chapter 9), who gives an historical and personal account of his long experience of being involved with psychiatry.

In order to arrive at a more democratic and fair position in relation to patients, practitioners might reflexively consider how their past and current personal and professional experiences, class, gender, race, ethnicity and age, create barriers in relation to hearing the stories of those who, perhaps ill advisedly, surrender their fate to the professionals. They might consider how the professional culture in which they live, in locating madness within the individual, creates a treatment barrier (Scott, 1973) in relation to productively including network of significant relationships in treatment (Reed, see Chapter 11). Reed goes on to argue that delimiting the individual as a unit of therapeutic intervention, leads to closure (Scott and Ashworth, 1967). The relatives of those diagnosed withdraw in order to protect themselves from hurt and pain. Such an analysis could even be shared with the clients themselves. This would allow the person in distress to weigh the advice given by the professional network against the possible prejudices that underpin that advice. It would expose what Boyle (Chapter 5) describes as 'therapeutic law', which works on the basis of professional discretion, to scrutiny. In reflecting team process (see Andersen, 1990, for a review) there is a detachment from the secrecy which professionals often maintain. For example, pre- and post-session staff discussions are infrequent, as issues are aired with the family. Andrews *et al.*, in their conference presentation reprinted as Chapter 10 of this book, offer a view from in front of the one-way screen on how they have dealt with the customary accoutrements to, and rituals of, working with families, which they argue are technologies of power.

EMPOWERMENT, LANGUAGE AND SOCIAL POETICS

There is a paradox of empowerment (Baistow, 1994). As it is currently conceived of, empowerment involves professionals giving back power to the laity in psychiatry. Price and Mullarkey define empowerment as 'The process of helping the client achieve a position or equality of power within the nurse/client relationship. . .' (1996: 17).[2] The application of Derrida's (1978) deconstructive enquiry is useful in this context. Deconstruction, as I interpret it, is a means of uncovering the conflicts within texts, and deciphering some of their multiple meanings. When the 'rules' of a text are applied to itself, deconstruction happens. As the act of giving back power is itself a powerful act – deconstruction happens. Perhaps the paradox of empowerment occurs because of a lack of an empowering language. Baistow (1994) notes that although the language used by 'empowerers' may have a radical tenor, e.g., a discourse of injustice, the empowerers resort to orthodox, individualizing psychology, e.g., counselling people about how to come to terms with the injustice they face. In the light of existing grammars of difference, e.g., diagnosis, the habits of practice are difficult to break. The great divide between knower and known, between health and welfare professional and users/clients/ patients is perpetually re-enacted. Even when, as Ron Coleman (Chapter 4) describes, service user involvement in planning is initiated, 'tame' user representatives are involved who do not upset the status quo.

Social poetics (Shotter, 1998) may offer a way of bypassing the production of another language. In any case, who would develop and own such a language? What would it consist in? In the place of interaction dominated by professional monologue, Shotter (1998) suggests a dialogical approach to human relations. In this we would become sensitive to the response that others call out from us and not simply to 'self-talk' as data which we use as an indication of some inner state or towards an explanatory theory, in this case of psychiatric distress. As Bakhtin puts it:

> With a monologic approach (in its extreme or pure form) *another person* remains wholly and merely an *object* of consciousness, and not another consciousness. No response is expected from it and could change anything in the world of my consciousness. Monologue is finalised and deaf to the other's response, does not expect it and does not acknowledge in it any decisive force. Monologue manages without the other ... (1984: 292–3; original emphasis)

Seikkula *et al.* (1995) recommend a move from monologue to dialogue in treatment systems in order to increase their democracy. The first rule in dialogical communication is that the subject and object dichotomy is removed. Every participant is involved in a process of co-evolution. Change does not have to follow the formula: therapist brings about change in client. As Seikkula *et al.* see it:

> In a consultation with a physician, only the physician has the possibility to determine the actual meaning of the symptoms the patient describes. Unfortunately, the interview with the psychiatrist also often takes this form, because the psychic symptoms or other problems create an internalized sense only on the doctor's side when the doctor has the diagnostic map inside his/her head. The psychiatrist could change this monological context by commenting personally on the answers of the patient ... When monological utterances are used, they do not gain any internal meaning or understanding ... (1995: 66)

Jackson and Stevenson (forthcoming) have studied the positions which psychiatric nurses can adopt in relation to patients, and the social distance, kinds of knowledge and power that these positions entail. Respondents in the study (people from different psychiatric disciplines, service users and their families) all thought that nurses do, and/or ought to:

- veer towards being the patient's friend
- have the most intimate knowledge about the patient
- engage with the patient in 'ordinary' conversation

- become powerful in a non-coercive way, through caring with the patient rather than for her/him. (In his contribution to this book, Ron Coleman makes this self-same distinction.)

In moving towards a different level of understanding, Shotter (1998) urges professionals to re-engage with poetic forms of talk, those which are non- or pre-disciplinary. To be able to talk (and relate, for the two now converge) in this way will allow us a different level of understanding of the unique worlds and inner lives of those we meet with, and them a greater access to ours. In order to illustrate social poetics in practice, Shotter (1998) uses the case of Dr P (the man who mistook his wife for a hat) made famous by Oliver Sacks (1985):

> Presented by Sacks with a glove, and asked 'What is this?', he described it thus: 'A continuous surface . . . infolded in on itself. It appears to have . . . five outpouchings, if this is the word' (1985, p. 13). He could match it to an abstract schema, but he did not know how to 'go on' with it: he saw no relationship between it and a hand. Only later, when by accident he got it on, did he exclaim 'My God, it's a glove!' Previous to that point, even when prompted by being asked if it might fit or contain a part of his own body, he was quite unable to identify it. (Shotter, 1998: 41)

Shotter (1998) interprets this as Dr P being relationally unmoved by the objects in his environment. He could not link himself to his surroundings. However, Sacks (1985) noticed that connectedness was achieved by using alternative sensory channels and performances. For example, Sacks (1985) noted that Dr P could 'relate' to coffee and cakes by moving the plates in a musical rhythm. When the rhythm was interrupted, he was lost as to what the task in front of him was, but when his wife poured him some coffee he responded to the smell and 'he became related to his circumstances again' (Shotter, 1998: 42). Sacks (1985) attributed Dr P's reconnection to the world as being due to inner body music. This was used also to recognize others. Hence, Dr P would say 'That's Karl, I know his body music' (Sacks, 1985: 17). There are some memorable examples in common parlance of alternative ways of making sense of the world: smelling fear; tasting victory; the roar of the greasepaint, the smell of the crowd; singing a rainbow, etc.

Sacks (1985) was aware that seeing Dr P in a sterile clinical environment and making standard psychological assessments was not revealing anything of the person. Such structures and procedures stand in the way of a deeper level of comprehension. In order to gain a greater understanding of Dr P, Shotter (1998) points out that Sacks had to pay attention to what aspects of Dr P's behaviour were emotionally moving; to Dr P's way of relating to him; to contrasts and comparisons within interesting episodes; to talk about the 'case' in the first person and in a discursive style, rather than in the dry tone of much academic writing. In this he was practising social poetics. An example from psychiatric nursing research clarifies what social poetics can achieve. Aldridge (1998) undertook a phenomenological study of the meanings people attach to being labelled schizophrenic. One participant in the study, Beth[3], had been engaged at different levels within the psychiatric system (in-patient, community) and with different disciplines without benefiting from her veteran status in terms of being able to get on with her life as she wanted. On interview, it became apparent that Beth had re-authored her 'life after schizophrenia' by comparing herself frequently to Alice in Wonderland: 'I had a distorted body and my neck, and Alice's neck was distorted . . .' (Aldridge, 1998: 43).

Aldridge (1998) was excited and moved by the comparisons between psychiatric systems and Wonderland, which she pursued in the interview with Beth. She found that by applying the text of Alice within her research, she could reach a richer understanding of Beth compared with her previous clinical engagement. For example,

> When Beth was asked to define why she felt comfortable within the art room, she explained, 'If you don't want to talk or something, people know you're not feeling too good.' Beth compares her experiences to a night out in the company of her partner and his acquaintances. 'I just hated it . . . normal conversation,[4] laughing and joking on . . . I just couldn't cope with it.' Alice said, as she picked her way through the wood, 'At any rate I'll never go there again! . . . It's the stupidest tea party I was ever at in all my life!'. . . (Aldridge, 1998: 46)

In my view, Romme and Escher's (1993) approach to people hearing voices approaches the poetic. They are as interested in life history as in the voice hearing itself. This allows them to 'make sense' of the voice hearing experience without recourse to accepted diagnostic frameworks. Szasz, in this book, reminds us that one of the founding fathers of psychiatry, Bleuler (1911), knew that schizophrenic 'delusions' were meaningful. As Bleuler reports the statements of a schizophrenic patient, 'She says, "I am Switzerland." She may also say, "I am freedom," since for her Switzerland means nothing else than freedom' (1911: 429). Szasz is aware that Bleuler, whilst identifying schizophrenia as a disease, was also attuned to the idea that schizophrenic thinking was a form of poetry and protest.

Working with patients in a new, less power-loaded way, is not an easy matter for professionals. Boyle (Chapter 5) notes that challenging the scientific basis of diagnosis is socially threatening. We are then forced to re-visit the question of how to deal with madness. Aldridge (personal communication) was accused by the CPN involved with Beth's care of upsetting her, implying that this new way of talking was likely to cause a relapse (although none occurred). Seikkula *et al.* (1995) note that sometimes co-evolution in family meetings leads to unclear and confusing conversation and it is difficult for the team to engage in reflecting process. There is not a story that comes to life for the participants. However, the clinical effectiveness of other treatments within psychiatry is not evidenced beyond reasonable doubt. Alec Jenner, in his contribution, notes that the superseding of one neuro-transmitter theory with another indicates a flawed hypothesis. Masson (1989) has comprehensively criticized psychotherapies as dangerous to health rather than life-enhancing.

CONCLUSION

In the spirit of the post-modernist position from which I write, a single conclusion is *passé*. I want to allow for the usefulness of different languaging of mental illness. Perhaps my ending is best summarized by borrowing a quote from Szasz, presented later in this book:

> Some psychiatric critics – opposing the use of psychiatric drugs, electric shock treatment, or psychotherapy [and their incumbent language][5] – advocate the legal prohibition of these methods or relationships, on the ground that people need the protection of the state from the 'exploitation' intrinsic to the practice of psychiatry and psychotherapy. I regard coercive protection from psychiatric treatment as just as patronizing as coercive protection from psychiatric illness. Both are state-imposed denials of the basic human right to engage in, or refrain from, making contracts. (p. 53)

Contracts imply choice and negotiation . . . but those are stories for another time.

NOTES

1 My use of the first person is based on my reluctance to write a 'depopulated text' (Billig, 1992) which is devoid of myself as author in terms of my preferences, experiences, etc. which have made the writing the way it is. Secondly, the 'I' indicates a personal opinion that is not necessarily shared by other contributors to the book.
2 As an aside, I refer the reader to Shula Ramon's excellent chapter in this book that presents the problems that mental health workers have in their day to day struggle to engage in respectful partnerships with patients.
3 An alias given to protect confidentiality.

4 I take it that the 'normal' is as strange as the talk of Mad Hatters and March Hares. Ironically, the people in the art room are those who have been characterized as mad. Irony appeals to post-modernists.

5 My addition.

REFERENCES

Aldridge, D. (1998) *The Unique Singular Self*. Unpublished MSc Thesis, University of Newcastle.

American Psychiatric Association (1994) *Diagnostic and Statistical Manual of Mental Disorders*, 4th edn. Washington, DC: American Psychiatric Association.

Andersen, T. (ed.) (1990) *The Reflecting Team: Dialogues and Dialogues about Dialogues*. Broadstairs, Kent: Borgmann Publishing.

Anderson, H. and Goolishian, H. (1988) Human systems as linguistic systems: preliminary and evolving ideas about the implications for clinical theory. *Family Process*, **27**: 371–393.

Bakhtin, M.M. (1984) *Problems of Dostoevsky's Poetics* (ed. and trans. Caryl Emerson). Minneapolis: University of Minnesota Press.

Baistow, K. (1994) Liberation and regulation: some paradoxes of empowerment. *Critical Social Policy*, **14**: 34–46.

Balint, M. (1957) *The Doctor, His Patient, and the Illness*. London: Pitman Medical.

Bateson, G., Jackson, D.D., Haley, J. and Weakland, J.H. (1956) Towards a theory of schizophrenia. *Behavioural Science*, **1**: 251.

Billig, M. (1992) *Talking of the Royal Family*. London: Routledge.

Birch, J. (1996) Borderlines. *Journal of Family Therapy*, **18**: 285–288.

Birch, J. (1995) Chasing the rainbow's end and why it matters: a coda to Pocock, Frosh and Larner. *Journal of Family Therapy*, **17**: 219–228.

Birch, J. (1991) Towards the restoration of traditional values in the psychiatry of schizophrenias. *Context*, **8**: 21–26.

Bleuler, E. (1911) *Dementia Praecox, oder Gruppe der Schizophrenien*. Leipzig: Franz Deuticke.

Bruner, J. (1990) *Acts of Meaning*. Boston, MA: Harvard University Press.

Crawford, P., Nolan, P. and Brown, B. (1995) Linguistic entrapment: medico-nursing biographies as fictions. *Journal of Advanced Nursing*, **22**: 1141–1148.

Cronen, V. and Lang, P. (1994) Language and action: Wittgenstein and Dewey in the practice of therapy and consultation. *Human Systems*, **5**: 5–43.

Deleuze, G. (1969) *Logique du sens*. Paris: Éditions de Minuit.

Deleuze, G. and Guattari, F. (1988) *A Thousand Plateaux*. London: Athlone.

Deleuze, G. and Guattari, F. (1984) *Anti-Oedipus, Capitalism and Schizophrenia*. London: Athlone.

Department of Health and Welsh Office (1983) Mental Health Act. London: HMSO.

Derrida, J. (1978) *Writing and Difference*. London: Routledge.

Foucault, M. (1976) *Birth of the Clinic*. London: Tavistock.

Fox, N.J. (1993) *Postmodernism, Sociology and Health*. Buckingham: Open University Press.

Gould, S.J. (1981) *The Mismeasure of Man*. Harmondsworth: Penguin.

Hannah, C. (1994) The context of culture in systemic therapy: an application of CMM. *Human Systems*, 5: 69–81.

Harré, R. (1998) *The Singular Self: An Introduction to the Psychology of Personhood*. London: Sage.

Jackson, S. and Stevenson, C. (Forthcoming) What do people need psychiatric and mental health nurses for? *Journal of Advanced Nursing*.

Jenner, F.A., Monteiro, A.C.D., Zagalo-Cardosa, J.A. and Cunha-Oliveira, J.A. (1993) *Schizophrenia: A Disease or Some Ways of Being Human?* Sheffield: Sheffield Academic Press.

Horowitz, I.L. (1996) Thomas Szasz against the theorists. *Chronicles*, 3: 23–26.

Johnstone, L. (1994) Values in human services. *Care in Place*, 1: 3–8.

Laing, R.D. (1960) *The Divided Self*. Harmondsworth: Penguin.

Masson, J. (1989) *Against Therapy – Warning: Psychotherapy May Be Hazardous to Your Mental Health*. London: Collins.

Price, V. and Mullarkey, K. (1996) Use and mis-use of power in the psychotherapeutic relationship. *Mental Health Nursing*, 16: 16–17.

Reed, A. (1996) Economies with 'the truth': professionals' narratives about lying and deception in mental health practice. *Journal of Psychiatric and Mental Health Nursing*, 3: 249–256.

Romme, M.A.J. and Escher, A.D.M.A.C. (1993) Hearing voices. *Schizophrenia Bulletin*, 15: 209–216.

Sacks, O. (1985) *The Man Who Mistook His Wife For His Hat*. London: Duckworth.

Seikkula, J. (1995) From monologue to dialogue in consultation with larger systems. *Human Systems*, 6: 21–42.

Seikkula, J., Aaltonen, J., Alakare, B., Haarakangas, K., Keränen, J. and Sutela, M. (1995) Treating psychosis by means of open dialogue. In: S. Friedman (ed.), *The Reflecting Team in Action*. New York: Guilford.

Schneider, K. (1959) *Clinical Psychopathology*. (trans. M. Hamilton). London: Grune and Stratton.

Scott, R.D. (1995) *The Barnet Crisis Service*. Paper delivered at the 25th anniversary meeting of the Barnet Crisis Service.

Scott, R.D. (1973) The treatment barrier: Part 1. *British Journal of Medical Psychology*, 46: 45–55.

Scott, R.D. and Ashworth, P.L. (1967) 'Closure' at the first schizophrenic breakdown: a family study. *British Journal of Medical Psychology*, 40: 109–145.

Shotter, J. (1998) Social construction as social poetics: Oliver Sacks and the case of Dr P. In: B.M. Bayer and J. Shotter (eds), *Reconstructing the Psychological Subject: Bodies, Practices and Technologies*. London: Sage.

Stevenson, C. and Beech, I. (1998) Playing the power game for qualitative researchers: the possibility of a post-modern approach. *Journal of Advanced Nursing*, 27: 790–797.

Stevenson, C. and Reed, A. (1996) Guest editorial. *Journal of Psychiatric and Mental Health Nursing*, 3: 215–216.

Stewart, K., Valentine, L. and Amundsen, J. (1991) The battle for definition: the problem with (the problem). *Journal of Strategic and Systemic Therapies*, 10: 21–31.

Szasz, T. (1996) 'Audible thoughts' and 'speech defect' in schizophrenia – a note on reading and translating Bleuler. *British Journal of Psychiatry*, **168**: 1–3.

Szasz, T. (1993) *A Lexicon of Lunacy*. London: Transaction publishers.

Webb, C. (1992) The use of the first person in academic writing: objectivity, language and gatekeeping. *Journal of Advanced Nursing*, **17**: 747–752.

Wittgenstein, L. (1953) *Philosophical Investigations* (trans. G.E.M. Anscombe). Oxford: Blackwell.

Wittgenstein, L. (1980) *Culture and Value* (trans. P. Winch). Oxford: Blackwell.

Part One

Keynote presentations at the
Longhirst Hall Conference

Introduction

Phil Barker and Chris Stevenson

The chapters in Part One are edited versions of papers given by the keynote presenters at the Longhirst Hall Conference. Those keynotes brought together, for the first time, some of the most distinguished names in psychiatry, psychology and social work, complemented by a single, but powerful, voice from the user movement in the UK. Although all had a keen interest in the critique of psychiatric power and authority, their different emphases and, sometimes, clear disagreements with one another, were developed in their papers. This celebration of diversity was, arguably, the highlight of the conference. We hope that the light of diversity will shine through here, to illuminate and stimulate the reader.

It is self-evident that psychiatry has had, and must continue to have, a degree of power and authority. Were these attributes to be artificially removed, this field of human enquiry would be rendered toothless: no more could we 'chew over' the assumed facts of the human condition; and there would be no chance of us 'spitting out' anything resembling wisdom at the end of the day. It remains doubtful, however, whether psychiatry has accomplished these aims to the satisfaction of all the players concerned – from the users of services and their families, through the myriad professional agencies, to politicians and the person in the street. What seems clearer is that even those who recognize – if not actually disapprove of – the power and authority inherent in the field, must continue to confront this twin-headed monster. Indeed, power and authority may be no more than dimensions of the field's conscience. The question appears to be not *if*, but *how* we exercise power; and *what* should be the basis of the knowledge that represents our authority?

It should not be forgotten either that we are talking, specifically, about *psychiatric* power and authority. Although we talk glibly, and simplistically, about *mental health* and its associated services, *mental illness* remains our focus, and *psychiatry* the broad church within which most of us worship. Since its emergence as a branch of medicine in the first half of the nineteenth century, psychiatry has been concerned with the protection and social control of people assumed to suffer from disorders of mental activity. Whether that protection and control was always in their best interests remains in dispute. Almost 20 years later, a wide range of disciplines has emerged as either allies of, or alternatives to, medicine. Arguably, the biggest stumbling block to collaboration between these various groups – or most trivial, depending on your viewpoint – is the vexed issue of diagnosis: determining *what*, if anything, ails the people deemed in need of psychiatric care and attention. It is almost universally accepted that there does exist a wide – indeed growing – range of people who need some kind of special care and attention, related to what Harry Stack Sullivan first described as their 'problems of living'. What is disputed, often hotly, is what we should call such people; and to what extent the traditional psychiatric system helps, or hinders, the process of resolving such problems. As a way out of confronting these questions, many professionals – and some service users – have tried re-shaping the psychiatric language. Increasingly, we exchange 'mental disorders' or 'mental illness' for 'mental health problems' – a somewhat dire expression which, of necessity, must embrace everything from occupational burn-out to suicidal despair. Some disciplines now refer, unselfconsciously, to themselves as 'mental health workers' – as if united, in the best socialist tradition, with their 'users', in the struggle against . . . what? Distress? Disease? Discrimination? Social disorder? Social exclusion? Given that some well-known writers from the user movement refer to their 'madness', perhaps the struggle, for what it is worth, is with plain, old-fashioned, *madness*!

These observations reflect the preoccupation with political correctness (PC), which may well be reaching the end of its shelf-life. Orwell will be one among many who is rotating beyond the grave at the sound of the English language being corrupted, as so many people struggle with so many words to 'mean what they say, without actually saying what they mean'. Meanwhile, many will be left thinking that these semantic issues have hardly touched those who have, for whatever reason, been left outside the language playground of late twentieth-century mental health (*sic*). Those who are in most distress today are the descendants of those who first required the original development of the institution of psychiatry. They may provoke, by the very nature of their human problems, the review of psychiatric power and authority that will influence the field for the good of all concerned – recipients and providers.

This first part of the book sets the scene for the necessary, and ongoing, critique of psychiatry. The chapters range across philosophical and legal issues, through a critique of the diagnostic process and racial stereotyping, to how we respond to psychiatric distress, and the roles of different disciplines in ensuring that such responses are, truly, in the best interests of the person and the family. All such concerns pivot, of course, around the experience of the person who uses the service – either willingly, or because the power of law determines that there is no option.

An early 'user' of modern-day psychiatry, John Perceval, remarked that:

> 'lunacy is like drunkenness – it releases powerful forces within, which can ultimately work for the good, so long as a man does not abandon his judgement.'

If a single thread weaves its way through these seven chapters, it is the recognition that what we now call 'mental health problems' may conceal a source of personal power, which may work, ultimately, for the good. Such good might prevail, not only for the individual, but also for those who make a genuine offer of help. To ensure that such offers are genuinely *powerful* and *authoritative,* we might recall that Perceval also recognized that: 'many persons confined as lunatics are only so because they are not understood'. We hope that the processes of reflection and self-examination to be found in these chapters are part of a wider search for the kind of understanding that Perceval found wanting. Should we ever gain some of that understanding, we might change not only the lives of those in need of psychiatric care, but also our own – all who choose willingly to offer it.

Introduction to Chapter 3

Thomas Szasz

by Phil Barker

Thomas S. Szasz is probably the most famous living psychiatrist. Over a forty year period, he has tenaciously, and consistently, presented a critique of the misuse of what he sees as a pseudo-science to deprive unusual or difficult people of their civil rights. Although he has been associated with 'Anti-psychiatry', and in particular with R.D. Laing, he occupied a wholly different position from Laing. Indeed, it hardly needs re-stating that Thomas Szasz has long occupied his own, unique position in twentieth-century psychiatry.

Thomas Szasz is presently Emeritus Professor of Psychiatry at the State University of New York Health Center, Syracuse, New York. It is worth noting that his position as professor, although a tenured one, was not a chair. He headed no department and has noted in interview that he never sought power over others – whether patients or colleagues.

Thomas Szasz first came to public prominence following the publication of an essay entitled 'The Myth of Mental Illness' in the *American Psychologist*, in 1960. The book that was modelled on that essay – *The Myth of Mental Illness: Foundations of a theory of personal conduct* – was published the following year, and established his reputation as a controversial writer on the nature of psychiatric disorders and their relationship to personal freedom. He has published 28 books and over 600 chapters, reviews and newspaper columns. As he approaches his eightieth birthday, he continues to travel the world, lecturing and giving interviews. He was awarded the prestigious *H.L. Mencken Award* on no less than three occasions, and is acknowledged widely for the quality, not only of his rhetoric, but also of his command of the English language. This is, perhaps, all the more remarkable, given that, when he emigrated to America at the age of 18, he did not know a word of English.

The breadth of Thomas Szasz's education, and interests, are evident in his chapter, which addresses 'The case against psychiatric power'. Here he draws on a range of authors to help explore, and frame, his case against the abuse of power in psychiatry. The reader will note one of

Professor Szasz's characteristics: his careful use of the language – taking care over definitions and ensuring that he says exactly what he means. These attributes are clearly endangered in a climate where buzzwords replace terminology and psychiatric terminology is used, inappropriately, as part of everyday parlance.

This chapter is drawn from the paper that opened the Longhirst Conference. A man who appeared much younger than his years, who exuded great charm and good humour, delivered it to a rapt audience. Professor Szasz came expecting to be challenged, and clearly enjoyed the mix of scholarly and down to earth debate which followed. His chapter offers both to the reader: an opportunity to reflect, carefully, on the key philosophical issues, and to consider their relevance for the world of practice.

3

The case against psychiatric power

Thomas Szasz

> To commit violent and unjust acts, it is not enough for a government to have the will or even the power; the habits, ideas and passions of the time must lend themselves to their committal. (Alexis de Tocqueville, 1981: 297)

Political history is largely the story of the holders of power committing violent and unjust acts against their people. Examples abound: Oriental despotism, the Inquisition, the Soviet Gulag, the Nazi death camps, and the American war on drugs come quickly to mind. Involuntary psychiatric interventions belong on this list.[1]

When de Tocqueville spoke of 'unjust acts' he was speaking as a detached observer, viewing state-sanctioned violence as an outsider. From the insider's point of view, state-sanctioned violence is, by definition, just. Prior to the passage of the Thirteenth Amendment, the Constitution of the United States endorsed involuntary servitude as a just and humane economic system. Today, people throughout the civilized world endorse involuntary psychiatry as a just and humane therapeutic system. Making use of the fashionable rhetoric of rights, a prominent psychiatrist describes adding the 'right to treatment' to the existing criteria of civil commitment as a 'policy more realistically and humanely balancing the right to be sick with the right to be rescued' (Traffert, 1996). Yet the fact that the psychiatrist can use force to impose the role of mental patient on a *legally competent* person against his will is *prima facie* evidence that he possesses state-sanctioned power. In 1913, Karl Jaspers[2] acknowledged the unique importance of this element of psychiatric practice. He wrote:

> Admission to hospital often takes place against the will of the patient and therefore the psychiatrist finds himself in a different relation to his patient than other doctors. He tries to make this difference as negligible as possible

by deliberately emphasizing his purely medical approach to the patient, but the latter in many cases is quite convinced that he is well and resists these medical efforts. (Jaspers [1913] 1963: 839–40).

The systematic exercise of power requires legitimation. Formerly, Church and State – representing and implementing God's design for right living – performed this function. Today, Medicine and the State perform it. W.H. Auden put it thus:

> What is peculiar and novel to our age is that the principal goal of politics in every advanced society is not, strictly speaking, a political one, that is today, it is not concerned with human beings as persons and citizens, but with human bodies . . . In all technologically advanced countries today, whatever political label they give themselves, their policies have, essentially, the same goal: to guarantee to every member of society, as a psychophysical organism, the right to physical and mental health. (Auden, 1968: 987)

So long as the idea of mental illness imparts legitimacy to the exercise of psychiatric power, the myriad uses of psychiatric coercions and excuses cannot be reformed, much less abolished. Hence, for those opposed to psychiatric power, the principal adversary is psychiatric legitimacy; power is merely its symbol, violence only its most visible manifestation. Before we turn to an examination of psychiatric power, let us get our bearings straight about the nature of power in general.

Power is usually defined as the ability to compel obedience. Its sources are force from above, and dependency from below. By force I mean the legal and/or physical ability to deprive another person of life, liberty or property. By dependency I mean the desire or need for others as protectors or providers.[3] 'Nature' observed Samuel Johnson, 'has given women so much power that the law has very wisely given them little' (Johnson, 1981: 172). The sexual control women wield (over men who desire them) is here cleverly contrasted with their legal subservience (a condition imposed on them by men).

Because the definition of power as the ability to compel obedience fails to distinguish between coercive and non-coercive means of securing obedience, it is imprecise and potentially misleading. For example, when Voltaire exclaimed '*Ecrazez l'infame!*' he was using the word '*l'infame*' to refer to the power of the Church to incarcerate, torture and kill people, not to the influence of the priest to misinform or mislead the gullible. The distinction I draw here is not novel, yet needs to be stated and restated. The American philosopher Alfred North Whitehead put it thus: 'The intercourse between individuals and between social groups takes one of these two forms, force and persuasion. Commerce is the great example of intercourse by way of persuasion. War, slavery, and governmental compulsion exemplify the reign of force' (Whitehead, 1961: 83).

I use the word 'Power' narrowly, to refer to the legally authorized exercise of force,[4] and use the word 'influence' to refer to obedience secured by money or other rewards or temptations.[5] The potency of power, symbolized by the gun, rests on the ability to injure or kill the Other; whereas the potency of influence rests on the ability to gratify the Other's desires. By desire I mean the experience of an (unsatisfied) urge, for example, for food, drugs or sex. The experience is painful, its satisfaction is pleasurable. The individual who depends on another person for the satisfaction of his needs (or whose needs/desires can be aroused by another), experiences the Other as having power over him. Such is the 'power' of the mother over her infant, of the doctor over his patient, of Circe over Ulysses. In proportion as we master or surmount our desires, we liberate ourselves from this source of domination.

The paradigmatic exercise of psychiatric power is the imposition of an ostensibly diagnostic or therapeutic intervention on a subject against his will, legitimized by the state as protection of the subject from madness and protection of the public from the madman. Hence, the paramount source of psychiatric power is coercive domination. Its other source is dependency, that is, the need of the powerless for comfort and care by the powerful. Involuntary psychiatric interventions rest on domination, voluntary psychiatric interventions on dependency. It is as absurd to confuse or equate these two types of psychiatric relations as it is to confuse or equate rape and mutually desired sexual relations. I oppose involuntary psychiatric interventions, not because I believe that they are necessarily 'bad' for patients, but because I oppose using the power of the state to impose psychiatric relations on persons against their will. By the same token, I support voluntary psychiatric interventions, not because I believe that they are necessarily 'good' for patients, but because I oppose using the power of the state to interfere with contractual relations between consulting adults[6] (Szasz, 1982).

When a person suffers – from disease, oppression, or want – they naturally seek the assistance of persons who have the knowledge, skill or power to help them or on whom they project such attributes. In ancient times, priests – believed to possess the ability to intercede with powerful gods – were the premier holders of power. For a long time, curing souls, healing bodies and relieving social-economic difficulties were all regarded as priestly activities.[7] Only in the past few centuries have these roles become differentiated, as Religion, Medicine and Politics, each institution being allotted its 'proper' sphere of influence, each struggling to enlarge its scope and power over the others.

The separation of Church and State represents a sharp break in Western political history. Although still paying lip service to an Almighty, the American Constitution is, in effect, a declaration of the principle that only the State (Government) can exercise power legitimately, and that the sole source of its legitimacy is the 'happiness of the people' insured by securing 'the consent of the governed'. Gradually, all Western states have adopted this outlook. The Argentinian poet and novelist Adolfo Bioy Casares satirized the resulting 'happiness' thus:

> Well then, maybe it would be worth mentioning the three periods of history. When man believed that happiness was dependent upon God, he killed for religious reasons. When man believed that happiness was dependent upon the form of government, he killed for political reasons. After dreams that were too long, true nightmares . . . we arrived at the present period in history. Man woke up, discovered that which he always knew, that happiness is dependent upon health, and began to kill for therapeutic reasons. (Bioy Casares, 1980: 7)

Among these therapeutic reasons, the treatment of mental illness occupies a unique place.

Human beings are intensely susceptible to two types of unpleasant experiences, anxiety-and-guilt and pain-and-suffering. Each is a virtually inexhaustible source of dependency, on soul-doctors, body-doctors, or both. Religion – providing myth and ritual – relieves people of anxiety-and-guilt and promises a tranquil eternal life in the hereafter. Medicine – providing diagnosis and treatment – relieves people of pain-and-suffering and promises a healthy and endlessly extended life on earth. How does psychiatry fit into this picture (Szasz, 1994)?

The practice of the branch of medicine we call 'psychiatry' began with the confinement of troublesome persons in madhouses. As a result, two symmetrical populations came into being: The kept, called 'madmen' or 'mad women' and the keepers, called 'mad-doctors'. During the eighteenth century, the idea of insanity and the institution of the insane asylum became established as important – indeed, socially indispensable – medico-legal concepts and methods of social control. Soon, law, medicine and popular opinion came to see the insane asylum as the proper place for housing persons authoritatively declared (diagnosed as) insane. Initially, few people were troubled by the fact that the situation of the insane in the asylum resembled the situation of the prisoner in jail. The philosophy of the Enlightenment undermined this complacency, projecting the idea of human rights onto the centre stage of Western history. Depriving mental patients of liberty had to be reconciled with society's ostensible devotion to human rights. This task was accomplished partly by conflating and confusing the concept of illness (a bodily condition) with the concept of incompetence (a 'mental' condition and legal concept-and-category [*non compos mentis*]); and partly by subsuming civil commitment under the rubric of the State's police power, that is, its duty to protect the public from 'dangerous' persons (lawbreakers). This dual justification of psychiatric power has remained essentially constant for almost 300 years.

A crucial moment in the legitimation of modern psychiatric power occurred in Central Europe during the early decades of this century.[8] Although initially psychiatry and psychoanalysis were distinct and separate enterprises, they soon merged into a union that proved to be fateful for the future of the 'mental health services' industry. This union was brought into being by the collaboration between Eugen Bleuler and Sigmund Freud and their followers.

Bleuler was born in 1857, in Switzerland. After a successful career in psychiatry, in 1889 he became the head of the famed Burgholzli, the public mental hospital in Zurich. Unlike most psychiatrists, Bleuler wanted to know his patients as persona. Realizing that the psychiatric dogma of his day was useless for that purpose, he looked to Freud's writings for help. By 1902, he had read *The Interpretation of Dreams*[9] and made three complimentary references to it (Ellenberger, 1970). Two years later he initiated contact with Freud, writing him 'that he and all his staff had for a couple of years been busily occupying themselves with psychoanalysis and finding various applications for it' (Jones, 1953–57, vol. 2: 30).

In his biography of Freud, Ernest Jones commented: 'Because of the increasingly prominent position Bleuler held among psychiatrists, Freud was eager to retain his support' (vol. 2: 72). Then, displaying his incomprehension of psychiatric history, he added: 'Unfortunately, this state of affairs [friendship between Freud and Bleuler] did not endure . . . His [Bleuler's] interests then moved elsewhere, from psychological to clinical psychiatry' (vol. 2: 119). This is wrong. Bleuler had always been a clinical psychiatrist; and he never relinquished his interest in the psychological understanding of patients and never renounced his appreciation of psychoanalysis. In 1907, replying to his critics, Bleuler wrote:

> I consider that up to the present the various schools of psychology have contributed extremely little towards explaining the nature of psychogenic symptoms and diseases, but that . . . psychoanalysis offers something towards a psychology which still awaits creation and which physicians are in need of in order to understand their patients and to cure them rationally . . . (Bleuler [1907], quoted by Freud [1914]: 26).

In 1925, in a letter to Freud, Bleuler put this point even more strongly: 'Anyone who would try to understand neurology or psychiatry without possessing a knowledge of psychoanalysis would seem to me like a dinosaur – I say "would seem" not "seems" for there no longer are such people, even among those who enjoy depreciating psychoanalysis!' (Bleuler [1925], cited in Jones, 1953–57, vol. 3: 117).

In his epochal work *Demential Praecox or the Group of Schizophrenias* (published in 1911), Bleuler courageously incorporated a psychoanalytic perspective in his interpretation of the behaviour of schizophrenic patients. The following example is illustrative. A woman patient declares that 'She is Switzerland.' Bleuler wrote: 'She says, "I am Switzerland." She may also say, "I am freedom," since for her Switzerland means nothing else than freedom' (Bleuler, 1925). The patient's 'symptom' reveals that she is protesting against her confinement: Bleuler's use of this example reveals that he recognized the legitimacy of her protest.

This is not the place to dwell on Bleuler's monumental work. Suffice it to note that although he defined schizophrenia as a 'disease [that] is characterized by a specific type of alteration of thinking, feeling, and relation to the external world,' ([1911] 1950: 150) his foregoing remarks show that he recognized that schizophrenic 'thinking' was a type of poetry and protest as well.[10] However, by pathologizing the schizophrenic's behaviour, Bleuler undermined that common sense judgement and the psychiatric response to it: The person incarcerated in the mental hospital was made to appear as a medical patient suffering from a disease; the psychiatrist incarcerating him was made to appear as a medical doctor treating a disease; and the power-relations between them were buried more deeply than ever.

At the same time, Bleuler – who was honestly seeking the truth – did not let the matter rest there. In 1919 – when his reputation as a psychiatrist was second to none in the whole world – he wrote a book, now virtually forgotten, that is largely a denunciation of psychiatric power. He wrote: 'Many a case of "latent" schizophrenia is diagnosed as total in all certainty. Never does it occur to the doctor to consider all the consequences: confinement of the patient to a mental institution, deprivation of civil rights, abandonment of his profession, etc.' (Bleuler [1919] 1970: 115). Who spoke of the civil rights of mental patients in those days? Not Freud. Not psychiatrists. But Bleuler did. In the final paragraph of his book on schizophrenia, commenting on 'the most serious of all schizophrenic symptoms . . . the suicidal drive,' he declared:

> I am even taking this opportunity to state clearly that our present-day social system demands great and entirely inappropriate cruelty from the psychiatrist in this respect. People are being forced to continue to live a life that has become unbearable for them for valid reasons; this alone is bad enough. However, it is even worse, when life is made increasingly intolerable for these patients by using every means to subject them to constant humiliating surveillance. ([1911] 1950: 488)

Bleuler must have felt more than a little guilty to have advanced so disingenuous a disclaimer. No one forces a person to become a jailer confining criminals, or a psychiatrist confining mental patients.

Notwithstanding the sloppy scholarship of many psychiatric historians, it is important to remember that Sigmund Freud was not a
psychiatrist. In late nineteenth-century Europe, the term 'psychiatrist'
meant a physician working in the public hospital system. Because Jews
were barred from employment in state-run bureaucracies, they could not
be psychiatrists and hence could not force people to be their unwilling
patients.

Not only was Freud not a psychiatrist, most psychiatrists viewed his
writings as inimical to psychiatry. For example, the prominent German
psychiatrist Franz von Luschan blamed 'Bleuler for his astonishing
behaviour in helping to promulgate the epidemic [i.e., psychoanalysis].'
Psychiatrists objected to Freud's writings not because he opposed
involuntary psychiatric interventions – which he unquestioningly supported. Instead, they disapproved of Freud's work because they wanted
to see themselves as physicians whose professional identity is firmly
anchored in neurology and neuropathology; and because they wanted to
see their patients as suffering from *bona fide* diseases, that is, bodily
abnormalities with physical causes independent of the sufferer's personal
history. By introducing a new set of disease-causative agents – namely the
patient's life-history (especially 'traumas' suffered during childhood) –
Freud spoiled this purely physicalistic conception of aetiology and
pathology.[11] At the same time, he reinforced the established social
prestige of psychiatry with the seemingly scientific prestige of psychoanalysis. The psychiatric profession now became like a mighty river,
formed by the confluence of two large tributaries – the state hospital
system (confining and caring for some of the injured and injurious
members of society in institutions), and the theory and practice of
psychoanalysis (offering a system of interpreting behaviour and counselling to non-institutionalized, fee-paying individuals). As a result psychiatric power became more impervious to criticism than ever.

Although I offer no new information concerning the collaboration
between Bleuler and Freud, the inference I draw concerning its impact on
the history of psychiatry is, I believe, novel. Historians of psychiatry and
psychoanalysis have overlooked how Freud's coveting the blessings of
psychiatry, combined with Bleuler's perceptive use of psychoanalytic
insights, re-enforced the legitimacy of the psychiatric enterprise, which
had always laboured under a cloud of scientific and civil-libertarian
suspicion. Herewith the evidence.

In 1914, in 'The history of the psychoanalytic movement', Freud wrote:
'A communication from Bleuler had informed me . . . that my works had
been studied and made use of in the Burgholzli . . . I have repeatedly
acknowledged with gratitude the great services rendered by the Zurich
school of Psychiatry in the spread of psychoanalysis . . .' (Jones, 1953–57:
119). What did Freud mean here by 'psychoanalysis'? Clearly, he could

not have meant that its subjects *must be voluntary clients,* an element that, nine years earlier, he identified as intrinsic to the practice of psycho-analysis. In 1905, Freud declared: 'Nor is the method applicable to people who are not driven to seek treatment by their own sufferings, but who submit to it only because they are *forced* to by the authority of relatives' (Freud, [1905]: 263–4; emphasis added). If so, psychoanalysis was even less applicable to people who were forced to submit to 'it' by the authority of policemen, judges and psychiatrists.

It is reasonable to conclude that, in reference to his alliance with the psychiatrists at the Burgholzli, Freud did not use the word 'psycho-analysis' to identify a *voluntary* relationship between a healer and his subject but rather a body of ideas associated with his name. This interpretation is supported by his remark that 'Jung successfully applied the analytic method of interpretation to the most alien and obscure phenomena of dementia praecox [schizophrenia], so that *their sources in the life-history and interests of the patient came clearly to light.* After this, it was impossible for psychiatrists to ignore psychoanalysis any longer' ([1905]: 28).

As we know, it was not at all impossible for psychiatrists to ignore psychoanalysis, if the term 'psychoanalysis' includes respect for *the current life-history and civil rights of the patient.* Indeed, Freud himself led the legions that joyously proceeded to ignore the most obvious life-historical event in the life of the schizophrenic patient, namely that a psychiatrist is depriving him of liberty. I have called attention elsewhere to Freud's glaring neglect of Schreber's incarceration. In 1976, I wrote:

> In his most famous study of schizophrenia, the Schreber case, Freud devotes page after page to speculations about the character and causes of Schreber's 'illness' but not a word to the problem posed by his imprisonment or his right to freedom. Schreber, who was 'psychotic', questioned the legitimacy of his confinement, and Schreber, the madman, sought and secured this freedom. Freud, who was a 'psychoanalyst', never questioned the legitimacy of Schreber's confinement, and Freud, the psychopathologist, cared no more about Schreber's freedom than a pathologist cares about the freedom of one of his specimens preserved in alcohol. (Szasz, [1976] 1988: 39)

The writer and literary critic Gabrial Josipovici reminds us that 'We do not decipher people, we encounter them' (Josipovici, 1988: 307). The psychiatrist's power over the patient negates the possibility of a humane encounter between them. Indeed, interpreted as a command, the rule that we should not decipher but encounter the Other violates the canons of psychiatry and the laws of the Therapeutic State. To remain a psychiatrist, the psychiatrist must view his client as a 'patient' afflicted with a dangerous 'mental disease,' and himself as a physician whose task is not only to treat mental diseases but also to incarcerate innocent patients deemed to be 'dangerous' and exculpate guilty patients deemed to be innocent by reason of insanity. No amount of semantic transfusion from the vocabulary of psychoanalysis can, or was intended to, alter these elementary facts of psychiatry, characteristic of twentieth century life in free and totalitarian societies alike.

I want to offer some additional observations concerning Freud's contributions to the enhancement and legitimation of psychiatric power. In 1914, in his essay 'On narcissism', Freud wrote: 'Patients of this kind [schizophrenics] ... Display two fundamental characteristics: mega-lomania and diversion of their interest from the external world – from people and things. In consequence of the latter change, they become inaccessible to the influence of psychoanalysis and cannot be cured by our efforts' (Freud, [1914b]: 74). Characterizing the schizophrenic as a person who, by turning away from 'things and people,' deprives himself of the benefits of psychoanalytic treatment is like characterizing the atheist as a person who, by turning away from God, deprives himself of the benefits of religious salvation. Instead of acknowledging that the schizophrenic's avoidance of the ministrations of a psychoanalyst is a decision, similar to a person's decision to avoid the ministrations of a chiropractor or Christian Science healer, Freud defined it as itself a symptom of schizophrenia and implied that if the schizophrenic were willing to submit to the analyst, psychoanalysis could cure him.

Although psychiatrists as well as psychoanalysts now treat psycho-analysis as a branch of psychiatry, the truth is that before psychoanalysis was absorbed into psychiatry, the two enterprises were almost antithet-ical. Politically, the essence of the psychoanalytic relationship was the absence of coercions (traditionally present) in relations between psychia-trists and mental patients. Practically, this meant that the analyst's failure to respect the patient's personal autonomy and/or his interference in the client's life were incompatible with the psychoanalytic relationship. The respective aims, values and practices of psychiatry and psychoanalysis may be summarized as follows:

- To effect a cure, the psychiatrist coerces and controls his 'patient': he incarcerates the (involuntary) victim and imposes various unwanted chemical and physical interventions on him.
- To conduct a dialogue, the psychoanalyst contracts and cooperates with his 'patient': he listens and talks to his (voluntary) interlocutor, who pays for the services he receives. (Szasz, [1965] 1988)

Before psychoanalysis became institutionalized as a profession, the psychoanalytic relationship represented a genuinely new social develop-ment, namely, a non-coercive, secular help ('therapy') for problems in living (called 'neuroses'). The term 'psychoanalysis' then denoted a confidential dialogue between an expert and a client, the former rejecting the role of custodial psychiatrist, the latter assuming the role of responsible, voluntary patient. The psychiatric and psychoanalytic enterprises were thus based on totally different premises and entailed mutually incompatible practices.

● The traditional psychiatrist was a salaried physician who worked in a mental institution; his source of income was the state; he functioned as an agent of his bureaucratic superiors and the patient's relatives. The typical mental hospital inmate was a poor person, cast in the patient role against his will, housed in a public mental hospital.
● The traditional psychoanalyst was a self-employed professional who worked in his private office; his source of income was his patient; he functioned as his patient's agent. The (typical) analytic patient was a rich person (usually wealthier than the analyst), cast in the patient role by himself, living in his own home or wherever he pleased.

As soon as Freud achieved the recognition he craved, he destroyed the core value of the psychoanalytic relationship. I refer to his assuming the authority of certifying competence in psychoanalysis and requiring that individuals seeking to become psychoanalysts undergo a so-called 'training analysis'. If voluntariness is an essential element of the psychoanalytic relationship, then a compulsory training analysis is a contradiction of terms.[12] The betrayal of confidentiality intrinsic to training analysis drove a stake through the heart of the role of the psychoanalyst. The result was the destruction of the moral integrity and healing potential of the human encounter called 'psychoanalysis'.

For more than forty years I have argued that the institution of psychiatry rests on civil commitment and the insanity defence and that each is a paradigm of the perversion of power. If the person called 'patient' breaks no law, he has a right to liberty. And if he breaks the law, he ought to be adjudicated and punished in the criminal justice system. It is as simple as that. Nevertheless, so long as conventional wisdom decrees that the mental patient must be protected from himself, that society must be protected from the mental patient, and that both tasks rightfully belong to a psychiatry wielding powers appropriate to the performance of these duties, psychiatric power will remain unreformable.

Of course, many people do threaten society: they assault, injure, rob and kill others. Some are regarded and managed as criminals, others as mental patients. In either case, society needs protection from the aggressors. What does psychiatry contribute to the management of such persons? Civil commitment and the insanity defence: inculpating the innocent and exculpating the guilty. Both interventions authenticate as 'real' the socially useful fictions of mental illness and psychiatric expertise. Both create and confirm the illusion that we are coping wisely and well with vexing social problems, when in fact we are obfuscating and aggravating them. Alas, psychiatric power thus corrupts not only the psychiatrists who wield it and the patients who are subjected to it, but the community that supports it as well.

As Orwell's nightmarish vision of *Nineteen Eighty-Four* nears its climax, O'Brien explains the functional anatomy of power to Winston thus:

> No one seizes power with the intention of relinquishing it. Power is not a means; it is an end. One does not establish a dictatorship in order to safeguard a revolution; one makes the revolution in order to establish the dictatorship. The object of persecution is persecution. The object of torture is torture. The object of power is power. Now do you begin to understand me? (Orwell, 1949: 266)

The empire of psychiatric power is more than three hundred years old and grows daily more all-encompassing. But we have not yet begun to acknowledge its existence, much less to understand its role in our society.

NOTES

1 Unless the context calls for a restricted use of the words 'psychiatry' and 'psychiatrist', I use these terms to refer to all mental health professions and professionals.
2 Jaspers later abandoned psychiatry for philosophy.
3 The spheres of legitimacy for power and dependency, respectively, are defined by law, custom and tradition.
4 The legally unauthorized use of force is a felony.
5 The symbol of power (coercion) is the gun, of influence (power without coercion), money.
6 Some psychiatric critics – opposing the use of psychiatric drugs, electric shock treatment, or psychotherapy – advocate the legal prohibition of these methods or relationships, on the ground that people need the protection of the state from the 'exploitation' intrinsic to the practice of psychiatry and psychotherapy. I regard coercive protection from psychiatric treatment as just as patronizing as coercive protection from psychiatric illness. Both are state-imposed denials of the basic human right to engage in, or refrain from, making contracts.
7 Jesus and Mother Teresa still project this sort of image.
8 A further legitimation of psychiatric power occurred in the 1950s with the introduction of antipsychotic drugs. It is now re-enforced by brain scanning methods allegedly demonstrating that mental diseases are brain diseases that, nevertheless, ought to be treated by psychiatrists rather than neurologists.
9 *The Interpretation of Dreams* was published in 1900, the watershed date in the history of psychoanalysis.

10 The points I wish to emphasize here are, first, that thinking, feeling and relating to the external world are, *prima facie*, not matters of medical concern; and second, that whatever an 'alteration of thinking and feeling' might be, it is patently an inadequate justification for depriving a person of liberty.

11 Depending on one's point of view, one might also say that Freud improved these concepts. In any case, by adding psychogenesis to somatogenesis, and psychogenic diseases (for example, perversions) to somatogenic diseases (for example, pneumonia), Freud expanded the conceptual categories of aetiology and pathology.

12 Because children are, by definition, involuntary subjects, child analysis is also a contradiction of terms.

REFERENCES

Note: *The Standard Edition of the Complete Psychological Works of Sigmund Freud,* translated and edited by James Strachey (24 vols). London: Hogarth Press, 1953–1974 is hereafter cited as *SE*.

Auden, W.H. ([1962] 1968) *The Dyer's Hand, and Other Essays*. New York: Vintage, p. 87.

Bioy Casares, A. (1998) Plans for an escape to Carmelo. *New York Review of Books*, 10 April, p. 7.

Bleuler, E. (1925) Letter to Sigmund Freud, 17 February 1925. Cited in E. Jones (1953–57) *The Life and Works of Sigmund Freud*, vol. 3, p. 117.

Bleuler, E. ([1919] 1970) *Autistic Undisciplined Thinking in Medicine and How to Overcome It*, translated and edited by Ernest Harms, with a preface by Manfred Bleuler. Darien, CT: Hafner Publishing, p. 115.

Bleuler, E. ([1911] 1950) *Dementia Praecox or the Group of Schizophrenias*, translated by Joseph Zinkin. New York: International Universities Press.

Bleuler, E. (1970 [1914]) quoted in Freud, S. On the history of the psychoanalytic movement, *SE*, vol. 14, p. 26.

Clarke, W.R. (1980) *Freud, The Man and the Cause*. London: Jonathan Cape and Weidenfeld & Nicolson.

Ellenberger, H.F. (1970) *The Discovery of the Unconscious*. New York: Basic Books.

Freud, S. [1905] On psychotherapy, *SE*, vol. 7, pp. 263–264.

Freud, S.[1914a] On the history of the psychoanalytic movement, *SE*, vol. 14, pp. 26–27.

Freud, S. [1914b] On narcissism: An introduction, *SE*, vol. 14, p. 74.

Jaspers, K. ([1913]1963) *General Psychopathology*, 7th edn, translated by J. Hoenig and M.W. Hamilton. Chicago: University of Chicago Press.

Johnson, S. (1981) quoted in Auden, W.H. and Kronenberger, L. (eds), *The Viking Book of Aphorisms: A Personal Selection*. New York: Dorset Press, p. 172.

Jones, E. (1953–57) *The Life and Work of Sigmund Freud* (3 vols). New York: Basic Books.

Josipovici, G. (1988) *The Book of God: A Response to the Bible*. New Haven, CT: Yale University Press, p. 307.

Orwell, G. (1949) *Nineteen Eighty-Four*. New York: Harcourt Brace, p. 266.

Szasz, T.S. (1958) Psychoanalytic training: A sociopsychological analysis of its history and present status, *International Journal of Psychoanalysis*, **39**: 598–613.

Szasz, T.S. (1960) Three problems in contemporary psychoanalytic training, *A.A.A. Archives of General Psychiatry*, **3**: 82–94 (July).

Szasz, T.S. ([1976]1990) *Anti-Freud: Karl Kraus's Criticism of Psychoanalysis and Psychiatry.* Syracuse: Syracuse University Press, esp. pp. 136–137.

Szasz, T.S. (1982) The psychiatric will, *American Psychologist*, **37**: 762–770.

Szasz, T.S. ([1976]1988) *Schizophrenia: The Sacred Symbol of Psychiatry.* Syracuse, NY: Syracuse University Press.

Szasz, T.S. ([1965]1988) *The Ethics of Psychoanalysis.* Syracuse, NY: Syracuse University Press.

Szasz, T.S. (1994) *Cruel Compassion: Psychiatric Control of Society's Unwanted.* New York: Wiley, ch.6.

de Tocqueville, A. (1981) quoted in Auden, W.H. and Kronenberger, L. (eds), *The Viking Books of Aphorisms: A Personal Selection.* New York: Dorset Press.

Traffert, D.A. (1996) Dangerousness (Letters), *Psychiatric News*, **31**: 14 (5 January).

Whitehead, A.N. (1961) *Adventures of Ideas.* New York: Free Press.

Introduction to Chapter 4

Ron Coleman

by Phil Barker

Ron Coleman may well be one of the most well-known figures in the British 'user' or 'survivor' movement. Some would say that Ron is an 'unforgettable' character – making an impact both by his physical presence, but also by the power of his verbal delivery. He also possesses a remarkable capacity to evoke strong emotions in his audiences – from tears of anger to tears of empathic sadness.

Ron Coleman's life has, by his own admission and description, been a colourful helter-skelter affair. He has an honours degree in politics, and also spent time in the army. His longest 'career' was spent going in and out of psychiatric hospitals, for more than a dozen years, most often under the controlling powers of the Mental Health Act, ending up like all too many others, severely disabled by neuroleptic drugs, on his own dark road to nowhere. His encounter with Marius Romme and Sondra Escher was to turn that life around and Ron was to become one of the most articulate and powerful advocates for the Hearing Voices Network, which emerged from Marius and Sondra's pioneering work in Holland.

Ron Coleman may always have been something of a political animal, but he gained a new political edge when he found his own 'voice' as the national co-ordinator of the Hearing Voices Network in 1991. This was the beginning of a period of sustained creative output – writing, speaking engagements and fostering other 'voices'. He is an articulate, funny, disarming, iconoclastic raconteur, who peppers his stories with historical anecdote, and the puncturing of many a psychiatric ego. He has cultivated a wide network of companions – some would say fellow travellers – who share his political perspective. He has noted that, although people refer to him as a 'user activist' or 'survivor activist', he would like to reject both of these notions, in favour of just describing himself as 'Ron Coleman'. He says that his politics are simple: he is a revolutionary socialist, though he is not a member of any political party. By conviction, he is a Marxist Trotskyist, and he believes that only through revolutionary activity will the system be changed. He is fervent in his belief that there exists a 'duty' to fight for reform in the 'here and now'. He acknowledges that his publications – he began with friends and colleagues his own publishing house – are unashamedly political in that sense, aiming to reform psychiatry and its services, here *and* now.

Although there were other user speakers at the Longhirst Conference, Ron Coleman was the user keynote, and served his constituency well. His paper, which is edited here, was presented without notes – Ron pacing the dais rhythmically, building his peripatetic philosophy from his own stories of treatment and institutionalization, woven through his damning critique of the pseudo-science of psychiatry. Although such a performance can hardly be replicated, not least on the printed page, the values and the morals emerge here unscathed from the editor's pen. This is a man who, by his own admission, gave up his victim status. In so doing he has set other wheels spinning.

4

The politics of the illness

Ron Coleman

Fourteen years ago I was diagnosed as schizophrenic; five years ago that was changed to chronic schizophrenia; three years ago I gave that up and went back to being Ron Coleman.

The conference is about the 'Construction of Psychiatric Authority'. My first remit was to do something on the 'Politics of Experience', my second remit was to do something on the 'Politics of the Illness' around hearing voices. Instead, I'm not going to do either. I'm actually going to construct, or deconstruct and probably reconstruct this whole idea of 'Psychiatric Authority'. I have some different beliefs to a lot of people about what psychiatric authority is and why we have it.

Within schizophrenia, for instance, we are either (as I was called) made axe wielding and crazy or we are pathetic creatures that need people's help. I reject both notions. We are basically people, but we are never recognized as people. We are never treated with humanity, we are never treated as individuals, we are treated as a label.

Because, if you think of it: what is the major cause of schizophrenia? The cause of schizophrenia is simply the psychiatrist's pen. When he writes on a piece of paper *'schizophrenic'* he has produced a schizophrenic, so that is the fundamental cause of schizophrenia. Nothing else.

Today we root schizophrenia in all sorts of things. Some people root it in the family; some people root it in biology; some people root it in your genes. It's all nonsense. If you want to root schizophrenia in anything you root it in society because society needs schizophrenia. We need Fred and Rosemary West to be mad. We need the Yorkshire Ripper to be mad. We need Adolph Hitler to be mad. Because if they're not mad then we have all got the potential to be exactly the same. Society needs schizophrenia. Society needs madness. And therein lies the 'Construct of Psychiatric Authority' – society's need. I take a different political perspective from a lot of people because I'm a Marxist Trotskyist and I'm unashamed about that.

We heard a poet at the beginning of this conference, and I'm going to quote (or misquote) a poet called Nathaniel Lee, who was incarcerated in Bethlem:

> They said I was mad.
> I said they were mad.
> Bastards. They outnumbered me.

And there is the construction of madness. The whole issue of psychiatric power and the construction of that power is crucial and yet there's an attempt now to turn it on its head to say it doesn't really exist. We sum this up in one word, 'empowerment'. That's the favourite buzz word: *'Let's empower the users.'*

So what do we do, us professionals – *'there's a bit of power for you, there's a bit of power for you, there's a bit of power for you . . .Right, I'll go home now it's five o'clock.'* The only people that we empower are the people that agree with us. Have you noticed that when we set up these committees now, you've got to have 'user representation'? But what happens? You get the tame user in. You don't invite <u>me</u> to committee meetings, do you know why? Because I read the papers before I go to committee meetings and I make notes about the things on it. They don't want me there because I'm not a yes man. Users are used like that and it is political usage, because the purchasers are saying: *'In order to get funding you've got to have user consultation, so we'll have user participation. Anybody that agrees with us can participate, if you don't agree with us, you're out.'* So what do we do? We let users sell out and we cause splits in the user movement because users are forced to sell out. And that is nothing new.

People have this idea that the user movement came along with Ronnie Laing in the 1960s and in the late 1950s with the foundation of MIND. Not at all. The user movement started 376 years ago in this country when a petition was sent to the House of Lords from the poor distracted people of Bethlem, people who had been incarcerated by the system. They complained about physical restraints and treatments, about having to perform for their allowances for food, about their environment and poor food generally. That was what their petition was about. Then last year the users had another petition in MIND's Breakthrough Campaign, and do you know what we were complaining about? Physical restraints, chemical treatments, having to perform to get our DLA – we still have to perform! We still have to keep saying we're the 'chronic sick' to get benefits. And the food? Yes the food is still bad in hospitals. Nothing has changed in 376 years in the user movement – nothing. If anything, the oppression has got worse.

So, let's not call it 'Psychiatric Authority', let's call it what it is, it's an oppression against a group of vulnerable people in society. And it's a deliberate oppression – when we've got people like Margery Wallace from SANE, and the papers whipping up anxiety and anger against people like me. Everybody knows you're less likely to be killed by a psychiatric patient than you are by your own brother or sister. Percentage-wise, there's less chance of a psychiatric patient committing murder than any other group in society. A psychiatric patient is more likely to be murdered than to murder.

The problem is people don't even back us up. They turn around and say they believe in 'new ways of working'. Then they use all the same old arguments that the Nazi guards in the trials at Nuremberg used. 'I can not go against the orders of a psychiatrist.' It's exactly the same argument. It had no value then and has no value now. If you don't believe in what you're doing then you've got two choices: get out, or change it. Turning around and saying '*I can't go against my psychiatrist*' is not an excuse, it's not.

We talk about power as if users are powerless. Well, I've got news for you, we're not! Even when you've got us incarcerated, even when we're being injected, even when we're getting ECT against our will, we've still got power. It's the only power we've got left and it's the power they gave us, the power of our illness. The power to do what we like and blame it on the illness. That is power. You've all seen it haven't you, the madness in the ward? The pick up of the chair, the throwing of the chair through the window, the nurse running over and saying: '*Why did you do that?*' and the '*Do what? I don't know what you're talking about.*'

Going into the smoke room seeing everyone sitting there and just smashing the window – it really pisses them off. That's power, that's real power. And that's the only power we've got because you've denied us any other real power.

My favourite one for really pissing staff off was being 'specialized'. Because being specialized is a two-way thing. We can make it easy for them or we can make it hard depending on how we feel. Being specialized is probably one of the biggest invasions of a person's privacy. Two nurses go everywhere with you: it didn't matter where you went to – toilet, bath, bed, eating – they are there and you're sitting there saying, '*I don't like this, six weeks of being specialized and I've not masturbated.*' You know I'm human and I've got sexuality you know, or do you forget that? Mind you if I'm on some drugs I can't masturbate anyway because I lose any sexual desire. We never talk about these issues because we lose our sexuality the minute we walk into a hospital. We're not real people any more. You can't mention sex to a user. Look what happens when you find two users in bed together (and you do occasionally). You go in and you say stupid things like: '*What are you doing? What do you think they're doing!*'

So I'd be sitting there with the two nurses either side talking over me because they never talk to you when you are specialized, they just talk over you to each other. So I lead them a dance. I get up and walk over to the other side of the room and they get up and they follow me, and I'd turn around and sit down and as soon as the nurses sit down you get up and go back across the room – back and forward, back and forward, back and forward. All day back and forward thinking that I'm really annoying them, not realizing that they're changing every half an hour. And then at the end of the day they're writing in my notes, '*Ron was really agitated today, perhaps he needs more medication.*' So, you can become the victim of your own fight back, you become the only casualty of your own war, a war against the system that on the surface looks like it can't be beaten. You maintain the victim status, you reinforce the illness model and why not, because they don't give us anything else. That's all this system has given us, the illness model and that's where our power is rooted as users.

Here's one of the classic examples you see happening all the time. Somebody kicks off on the ward. The first in there are the nurses that are liked – they're first in because they're not in the office, they're on the wards where they're meant to be. They never get hit, have you ever noticed that? The first one in never gets hit even though this person is really kicking off mad (or supposedly so). And they're standing there confronting this mad person, and this mad person is not hitting them and then the one they *don't* like comes out of the office eventually and gets kicked. Where's the madness? There isn't any madness. There might be badness but it isn't madness. It's our opportunity to get our own back – to get back at them.

Power is a funny thing because I believe there are certain elements to power that we need as users and I think professionals can help in the process. I think one of the first elements we need is knowledge. Knowledge is power. Without a doubt we need information. Information about the rubbish they're pumping into our bodies – full information on their side effects, information on what happens when you put two neuroleptics into some poor sod's body. We need that information because without that information we cannot start our fight-back. And our fight-back is based on that, based on knowledge. You can't fight back without knowledge because when you go back and say, '*I think there's something going on here,*' they say, '*That's all right, Ron, because you lack insight. It's part of your illness, Ron, thinking that there's something "going on". It's a delusionary process.*'

Knowledge would be a weapon that users could use, and actually *are* using now. We're gathering knowledge from around the world because we've finally learnt the value of networking. Something that professionals have been doing for years and we've finally cottoned on to it. As we gather this information together we're beginning to use it. Information that shows if you switch an ECT machine off we recover just as well as if an ECT machine was switched on! We're beginning to get our hands on the kind of information that's been denied to us and we're using it to challenge some of the things that our psychiatrists are doing.

Mental health professionals are agents of the State. Our Mental Health law is enshrined by Government. This means that mental health professionals have always got to cover their backs. That's the biggest risk they've got, isn't it? If something goes wrong, they will get the blame for it. So, yet again they dis-empower the user saying: *'He can't take responsibility for himself.'* They care for us, don't they? Come on, let's be honest, they don't go into this profession for the money do they? No, they go into this profession because they care for us. Well we don't want them to care for us. We want them to care about us. There's a difference. Because when you care *about* us you can take risks, but when you care *for* us you can't afford to take risks.

We do not want you to work *on* us any more. We want you to work with us and that means on our terms not your terms. And we don't want you to perceive our needs because this is what professionals do, they are wonderful at it: *'This person needs this, this, this and this.'* You never ask us what we need because the thing we need for power is money – you know 'brass', 'cash', the stuff you get for looking after us. We don't get any money and we need it because money is power – economic power.

I hate the Tories – and I hate Labour just as much because they've just become another bunch of Tories – but if you look at one thing that's happened because of the purchaser/provider split, users are beginning to get a voice, not a very big voice but a voice. I wish they'd go a stage further, I wish they'd turn around individual users and say: *'Here's your money. Now do with it what you like.'* The professionals would soon pull their socks up. We'd soon get choices that weren't heard of before.

In our country psychotherapy, for example, is given on the National Health Service. Even people that are psychotic and hear voices are given psychotherapy on the NHS – especially if you're middle-class and white. If you're working-class and black you don't get it. Because we're not articulate enough, us working-class people. We swear, we've got foul language and things. We can't articulate our problems but middle-class people of course can articulate their problems, so they can get it. We still live in a classist, racist, sexist, homophobic system. They may have said that homosexuality was no longer a mental illness in the 1970s but in a lot of places it's still treated as if it is. Gay people are not only oppressed within the system if they've got a 'mental illness' but also for the fact that they're gay as well.

Schizophrenia has a higher incidence rate amongst black people (and I'm just using the word schizophrenic because it does exist because psychiatrists say it exists and society says it exists). Schizophrenia has a 1 per cent incidence rate around the world. In Britain, however, if you're black then it's 10 per cent. If you go to a black country it's 1 per cent, in Britain it's 10 per cent. The reason they're giving for it at the moment is that it happens in the womb! It's a brain disease more common in black people who are immigrants. Of course it's nothing to do with the fact that we live in a racist society that attacks black people, that doesn't let black people have real jobs, that doesn't let people have a proper education – that doesn't play a part in it! It's the same if you're Irish in this country. Higher numbers of Irish people are sectioned. It's out and out racism and it's based on the power of the English Establishment. I use my words carefully – English Establishment.

So how can we get through this dilemma, how can we change these ideas and work together. The simple answer is we can't. On one level we simply can't work together. We will never be in partnership as equals so let's dump that notion that partnership talks about equality, because at the end of the day they will always fall back on the responsibility to care under common law because they are scared. Notice how many people get sectioned on Fridays: *'I'm going off for the weekend so I'd better get him sectioned then I know he'll be around on Monday.'* Have you thought about it? What power and what arrogance! Is that the construction of psychiatric power – while you're having a holiday you'd better get your client into hospital? That's the sort of nonsense we're subjected to day in, day out.

Never having been a voluntary patient, I had a thing about being a voluntary patient. If you went in voluntarily and you smashed a window you had to pay for it. So I always reckoned being sectioned was a safer bet because I used to enjoy smashing windows. There's no point in being a voluntary patient in this country; even voluntary status is an illusion. We say that people are voluntary patients and we don't mean that. If we don't try to walk out you won't give us your piece of paper saying we're sectioned. But to all intents and purposes voluntary patients are treated as people who have been sectioned. What power do we give these people? In Manchester, last time I was under section, I appealed and was told it would be twelve weeks before the tribunal would hear my case. In this country if you're arrested by the police you're up in court the next day (unless it's a Saturday night and then it's Monday). Normally they'll bail you anyway then. If you're arrested in this country for something like murder, they've either got to charge you within 72 hours or apply for an extension to the court to keep on questioning you. If you're arrested under the Prevention of Terrorism Act you must be brought before a judge within 10 days. If you're sectioned under the Mental Health Act you do not see your superiors for twelve weeks. What power! Is that not abuse? You know what they can do in those twelve weeks, especially if you get a second opinion. You can get a lot of neuroleptics pumped into your body in twelve weeks.

I think the very first campaign needs to be started in this country stating that if the person doesn't want treatment then no treatments are to be given until a tribunal has been held. Don't talk to me about manager's tribunals because it's just a load of accountants who don't know anything. They tend to put accountants on appeal tribunals where I live. What does he know about Mental Health? He's got a psychiatrist saying to him: *'If that guy goes out and tries to kill somebody it's your fault.'* I'm saying that they're making the decisions.

I don't believe it's just about people that hear voices any more – I think it's also people that see things, feel things, people that are mentally distressed. At the end of the day I don't believe in schizophrenia. I don't believe in mental illness any more because evidence doesn't stack up. There is no scientific evidence on schizophrenia, there's no lab tests. It's a subjective piece of work. It's something a psychiatrist gives you. We've got a theory about diagnosis in voice hearers (if you see a psychiatrist). If you've got a straight face you're schizophrenic. If you're smiling when you see him you're a manic depressive. And if he doesn't like you you've got a personality disorder. That's our theory around what is actually happening, and it is.

You get different diagnoses from different psychiatrists. You go to see three different psychiatrists with the same symptoms the chances are you'll get three different diagnoses depending on what the psychiatrists last read. That's a sad state of affairs, isn't it! But that's power.

To achieve real power, to deconstruct the power of psychiatry, I don't believe it can be reformed. I don't believe you can actually reform an establishment. I think what you can do is deconstruct an establishment and reconstruct something new, to put in place of that establishment. But for people like us to actually take a part in that battle we're going to have to change the way we've worked up until now. We're going to have to give up the idea that the way forward is somehow to petition the government or to think that the government is going to change things. We've got a government that thinks all the economic problems in the country are caused by single parents. How are they going to change things? The only reason they brought through the last bill on Mental Health is because they thought they'd get a few votes out of it, and all the political parties are the same. Mental Health is not a great vote winner unless its used to oppress people with mental distress. It's the only way to win votes out of Mental Health, not by empowering people, not by liberating people but by oppressing people. That is the only vote winner in Mental Health.

So we can't look to the government. So who can we look to? We can only look to ourselves, in the first instance, because at the end of the day you can give up being mentally ill. It's dead easy to give up, you just say 'I'm not mentally ill.' That's the first step. You reject the notions that you're ill. You might be distressed, you might have problems but you're not ill. Because look at the construction. Once you've got a diagnosis and you wake up in the morning you're down, sad or blue: then you're depressed because you have a diagnosis. You wake and you feel happy with the joys of spring, England won the other night, great, etc. I'm manic because I've got a diagnosis. I wake up and I'm angry, and if it's seen on the ward it's seen as aggression, it's part of my illness. I've got an illness and normally I'll be treated forcibly because somebody like me doesn't take medication. You lot can have hobbies, you can even be train-spotting and even that's called aspro syndrome. Yours are called hobbies, mine are seen as 'obsessions'. If you don't clean your house for a week, you're a lazy sod. If I don't clean my house for a week, I lack daily living skills!! A symptom of schizophrenia, I'm not a lazy bastard, I'm ill!! That's how it works. That's the nature of power. The power to oppress people.

We've got to do it in the same way as the gay movement. No longer should we hide behind the illness. We should stand up and use the illness as our power. I hear voices, I still hear voices, but that doesn't make me ill. It makes me psychotic and proud! That's what it makes me. I'm not ill, I've never been ill, I've been distressed but not ill. We've got to stand up and own our experience because the experience is not owned by psychiatrists, by nurses or social workers and it's not owned by your family. The experience of hearing voices can only be owned by the voice hearer and the same goes for any other mental distress.

It's only through ownership and giving up the victim status that you can begin to give up being a victim of the system. It's only then can you get on with your life. Ownership means taking responsibility for your own life. That's not easy, because when you take up responsibility you can't keep running back to the hospital every two minutes. Every time anything goes wrong you cannot blame an illness any more. It's about you and life because life is hard. We live in a hard world. We've lived through a hard system and if we can survive that system we can survive out there.

Introduction to Chapter 5

Mary Boyle

by Chris Stevenson

No discussion of power and authority in psychiatry is possible without a careful examination of diagnosis and classification, given their core function as both the definitions of what allegedly ails people with mental health problems, and also the rubric by which treatment is determined. I found no difficulty in deciding who should address these issues at the Conference, since Mary Boyle had already established a formidable reputation as part of her crusade against the inappropriate labelling and classification of people as 'schizophrenics'.

Mary Boyle knows much about the world of psychiatric practice, having been a clinical psychologist for more than fifteen years. Perhaps it is exactly that proximity to people, and their problems of everyday living, which has energized Mary Boyle's particular crusade. Certainly, her 1990 text on 'Schizophrenia: a scientific delusion' has excited opinion, throughout the psychiatric field. It is worth noting that this text is recognized as a piece of formidable scholarship, not least because it comes from within a discipline which has built its twentieth century reputation – at least in the Western world – on a science of human categorization.

Presently, Mary is Head of Clinical Psychology at the University of East London where she is responsible for the training programme in clinical psychology. It is worth noting that in her writing she refers to figures such as Foucault who, typically, are not part of the psychological canon. I presume, therefore, that she brings to her teaching a breadth of scholarship and provocation that perhaps all students deserve by right.

5

Diagnosis, science and power

Mary Boyle

I am concerned here with three aspects of psychiatric diagnosis. First, with the ways in which psychiatric diagnosis can be thought of as a form of power; second, with the relationship between science and diagnosis as a form of power and, third, with some of the obstacles to disempowering diagnosis. This last aspect is considered in the hope that it might provide pointers to the issues that need to be confronted in trying to disempower psychiatric diagnosis.

DIAGNOSIS AND POWER

Diagnosis is central to the practice of psychiatry and receiving a psychiatric diagnosis can have a profound impact on people's lives. Yet diagnosis is rarely presented, at least in the traditional accounts, as other than a neutral activity which involves the objective application of research findings and clinical judgement. The American Psychiatric Association's *Diagnostic and Statistical Manual of Mental Disorders*, for example, claims that it does not categorize people (which might not be seen as a neutral activity) but '[mental] disorders which people have' (1994: xxii). This claim helps create the impression that there exist 'out there' naturally occurring mental disorders and that the task of the diagnostician is simply to recognize and record their occurrence. Although it may be acknowledged that individual clinicians differ in their diagnostic acumen or that 'misdiagnosis' may occur, there is no place in this account for diagnosis to be seen as a *systematic* practice of power.

Foucault's (1979, 1980) theory of the relationship between language, knowledge and power will be used here to provide a framework for a strongly contrasting picture of psychiatric diagnosis. As Foucault pointed out, traditional models depicted power as an entity which could be seized or passed on; as a possession, as when we talk of people 'having power' or 'giving power to ...'. Within these essentialist or juridical models, power flows from a centralized source such as law or government and is mainly repressive or subtractive, i.e. it operates through sanctions, laws and prohibitions. Foucault did not suggest that this form of power was unimportant; rather, he argued that over the last two centuries or so, it had been superseded by forms of power whose operation was more subtle and obscure. Foucault used the term 'bio-power' to convey the idea of power over bodies and minds; as Sawicki (1991) has noted, bio-power emerges as 'an apparently benevolent but peculiarly invasive and effective form of social control' (1991: 67). Foucault described two related forms of bio-power. The first, a bio-politics of the population, consists of a series of social and economic policies, interventions and laws relating to birth, marriage, death, health and reproduction. The second form of power, disciplinary power, is of particular interest in relation to psychiatric diagnosis.

Disciplinary power can be seen as operating in three major ways. The first is through language and its links to social practice. In this framework, language does not reflect reality; it *constructs* it; in effect it 'tells' us to see people and the world in particular ways and effectively disbars or obscures alternative visions. Thus, when the DSM claims to categorize 'mental disorders which people have', it brings into being a world which includes a pre-existing category of object called a mental disorder which can become a property or possession of the person. Not only that, but language is *strategic* in the sense that it may be used to achieve certain ends, to make certain courses of action seem appropriate and reasonable and others unreasonable or even unthinkable: to construct a world which contains mental disorders is to suggest that it is reasonable, even necessary, to discover and describe these and to identify those who are affected by them. And the term 'diagnosis', with its links to medical practice, appears to mandate certain actions towards those who receive a psychiatric diagnosis – the attention of health professionals, admission to hospitals, physical treatments – and to make other actions, such as contact with teachers or priests, seem less appropriate.

The second way in which disciplinary power operates is through the production of certain identities. Indeed, it was its productive nature which, Foucault claimed, most distinguished disciplinary power from subtractive forms of power based on sanctions and prohibitions. One of the major results of diagnosis has been to produce certain categories or types of people: there have always been children who won't sit still or do what their parents and teachers tell them; it is only recently that there have been children suffering from attention deficit disorder. There have always been women who prefer not to have sex with their husbands. Now we have a new type of woman who suffers from hypoactive sexual arousal disorder. And not only does psychiatric diagnosis produce new types of people, it does so at an alarming rate: the DSM-1 listed 106 diagnostic categories; DSM-II had 182; DSM-III had 205; DSM-IIIR had 292 and DSM-IV has 390 (Sarbin, 1996).

Disciplinary power operates, finally, through the creation of privileged ways of talking and writing about particular phenomena and the attachment of these practices to particular professional groups. The DSM draws on two highly privileged languages: those of science and medicine which operate to create a powerful impression of both care and concern and of objectivity and neutrality and whose effect is to discourage or deflect criticism or disagreement. An imbalance of power which is exceptionally difficult to challenge is therefore created between those who carry out the diagnostic process and those to whom it is applied.

Although it is difficult to overestimate the importance of disciplinary power in relation to psychiatric diagnosis, one of the results of Foucault's emphasis on it has been a de-emphasis of juridical or legal power. Discussing the role of gender in legal theory, Smart (1989) has criticized Foucault for failing to provide an adequate account of the relationship between disciplinary and juridical power and for underestimating the continued influence of the latter. The importance of such an analysis in relation to psychiatric diagnosis will be considered in the next section through a discussion of mental health legislation.

POWER AND MENTAL HEALTH LEGISLATION

Mental health legislation is a crucial area where juridical and disciplinary power come together, where the centralized power of the law to subtract, to sanction, to prohibit or to impose, comes together with the diffuse operation of disciplinary power in constructing and producing, and in using language for subtle forms of self and social regulation. The alliance of these two forms of power in mental health legislation will be examined through an important distinction between two types of law highlighted by Bean (1980): formal law and therapeutic or purposive law. Formal law governs criminal acts such as murder, assault, burglary and fraud, and has a number of important features. First, the state's role in formal law is as accuser and penalizer; there is no suggestion that the operation of the law is supposed to benefit the accused. Second, the law is interpreted and operated by the judiciary, by barristers, judges, magistrates and juries. Third, formal law usually operates in public: we may attend trials or read about them in the press or law reports. Finally, because formal law is not assumed to benefit its recipients, there are extensive provisions against its wrongful operation, such as the initial assumption of innocence, stringent standards of 'proof' and the right to defence or appeal. By contrast, therapeutic or purposive law, of which mental health legislation is an example, has quite different features. First, its emphasis is on protecting or enhancing the welfare of its recipients, so that the law is supposed to act for their benefit and in their interests. Indeed, the very term 'mental health legislation' or 'Mental Health Act' implies that achievement or maintenance of 'mental health' is the major aim of the legislation. Second, therapeutic law is usually operated not by the judiciary but by professionals and administrators because it is assumed that people other than lawyers or judges can best interpret the law. Third, the rules of therapeutic law are explicitly formulated to allow professional discretion in decision-making so as to take account of particular aspects of individual cases. Fourth, therapeutic law usually operates in relative privacy; full records of its procedures may not be kept and it may be difficult for the public to gain access to its workings. Finally, in contrast to formal law which gains its authority from adherence to formal procedures, appeals to precedence or to the rulings of higher law-making bodies, therapeutic law derives its authority from appeals to science or, at least, to specialist knowledge supposedly possessed by those professionals empowered to interpret and operate the law.

All of these features are crucial to the operation of therapeutic law and they are clearly interrelated; however, I want to highlight two: that therapeutic legislation is not operated by the judiciary and that it derives its authority from claims to be based on specialist scientific knowledge. It is, of course, *because* of this claim that the judiciary are willing largely to be excluded; it is also because of this claim that therapeutic law is seen as not requiring the safeguards of being subject to strict rules and procedures or of operating in public. The objectivity of scientific knowledge and the objectivity of those who apply it, are assumed to be sufficient safeguard.

We can see here the ways in which juridical and disciplinary power reinforce each other in the operation of therapeutic law. The law's reliance on the disciplinary power of knowledge allegedly gained through science, makes the law less public, less accountable and therefore more difficult to challenge. And the explicit incorporation of psychological and psychiatric knowledge into the law arguably strengthens that knowledge and makes it more difficult to challenge by giving it credibility well beyond the confines of textbooks and journals.

The claim to be based on scientific authority, or at least on secure specialist knowledge, is central to the operation of therapeutic law. A good deal of this claimed scientific basis to mental health legislation concerns psychiatric diagnosis, because the law is concerned with the identification, placement and management of those said to be suffering from treatable mental disorders, and these people are said to be recognized through the process of diagnosis. Diagnosis then, is doubly powerful: it functions as a form of disciplinary power by creating types of people who appear to exemplify natural categories of mental disorder; by defining social norms of behaviour and experience; by telling us how to think about people who deviate from these norms and by making certain forms of management seem desirable and appropriate. Diagnosis, however, also functions as a form of juridical power, through the law's reliance on the process. But how valid is the claim that diagnosis (and, therefore, mental health legislation), is based on scientific or secure specialist knowledge? Detailed discussion of this claim is beyond the scope of this chapter (see Boyle 1990, 1996) but an overview of the major issues will be given.

THE SCIENTIFIC BASIS OF PSYCHIATRIC DIAGNOSIS

These concepts of reliability and validity are fundamental to diagnosis. Reliability refers to the extent to which clinicians agree on the diagnoses that should be applied to particular people. There is a great deal of evidence that psychiatric diagnoses are unreliable (for example, Bentall, 1990; Kirk and Kutchins, 1992) and a great deal of effort has been expended in trying to develop diagnostic criteria which can be applied reliably. Indeed, the form which the DSM has taken since its 3rd edition in 1980, in which each diagnostic category is accompanied by a list of criteria for applying it, is part of this process of trying to ensure reliability of diagnosis. All of this seems eminently sensible. After all, consistency has been a major value in science at least since the time of Francis Bacon. The problem with these efforts is that they make no sense scientifically because they completely misrepresent the relationship between reliability and validity as they apply to diagnosis. This point can hardly be overemphasized and needs to be made very strongly indeed because of the persistent emphasis on diagnostic reliability and efforts to improve it, and the de-emphasis of validity (e.g. Wing, 1988; APA/DSM-IV, 1994).

The importance of this relationship can be seen by considering two crucial aspects of diagnosis and the meaning of validity in this context will arise from the discussion. The first is that psychiatric diagnosis gains much of its credibility through the implication that it is the same sort of process as medical diagnosis. The second is that diagnosis is, or is supposed to be, a form of pattern recognition. What this means is that diagnosis is not an independent activity; it is, or should be, entirely dependent on prior successful research which has identified meaningful relationships amongst apparently disparate phenomena.

What happens in medicine, or is supposed to happen, is this: people complain of all sorts of physical maladies and examination of their bodies reveals all manner of phenomena which may or may not be related to their complaints. The potential number of complaints, or discoveries which may be made about body functioning, are enormous and the task of medical researchers is to make sense of these, to try to discover what goes with what, to describe regularities amongst complaints and bodily functioning. Of course, it is easy to see these relationships with hindsight – once we know that a genital sore is related to brain damage later in life (tertiary syphilis) or that high blood pressure is associated with kidney malfunction, the connections may seem obvious but it is not so easy with only foresight to go on; the task facing medical researchers may therefore seem far easier and less prone to error than it actually is.

There are various rules in medical research for trying to decide whether any hypothesized relationship amongst bodily phenomena is meaningful or illusory (see Boyle, 1990 for a detailed discussion). When researchers believe, rightly or wrongly, they have identified a meaningful pattern, they usually infer a concept, e.g. diabetes, leukaemia, multiple sclerosis, which becomes an heuristic or an aid to research. Much of this research is aimed at identifying underlying processes that are assumed to account for the 'surface' relationship between complaints and bodily functioning.

Diagnosis is the name given to the *secondary* process in which clinicians recognize new exemplars of these patterns which have already been identified by researchers. In other words, it is a process that is entirely dependent on previous research. So, when a clinician says: 'You have multiple sclerosis', what they are actually saying is that you show the same set of physical features previously shown by researchers to be meaningfully related; researchers inferred the concept of multiple sclerosis from this pattern and so I'm doing the same. We can also see from this that what we call diagnostic criteria are really a statement of the elements which make up this pattern of physical features which researchers have identified. And what we think of as a diagnostic label is actually a concept, an abstraction, inferred from that pattern. The idea of validity in relation to all of this means the extent to which this concept is useful in taking forward research that identifies the processes underlying these patterns. In other words, the validity of a diagnostic concept refers to its usefulness (and 'utility' is often used as another term for validity) in making new observations as, for example, when the concept of Down's syndrome proved useful in identifying previously unobserved chromosomal abnormalities. It is this capacity to generate new observations which helps convince researchers that their concept *is* derived from a meaningful pattern and not from a chance co-occurrence of unrelated phenomena. In this sense, then, the idea of validity applies only to the concepts inferred during the diagnostic process and not to any particular diagnosis: diagnoses themselves can only be described as more or less accurate, i.e. in terms of the extent to which the phenomena observed in the person who is given the diagnosis match those previously identified by researchers who inferred the diagnostic concept.

IMPLICATIONS FOR PSYCHIATRIC DIAGNOSIS

All of this has profound implications for psychiatric diagnosis. The process by which diagnostic concepts are, or should be developed by researchers means that there should be no need to search for reliable diagnostic criteria for particular diagnostic labels. The reason for this is that the concepts inferred during diagnosis should come ready equipped with the criteria for inferring them, as it is the existence of the pattern which the criteria describe, which justifies inferring the diagnostic concept in the first place. If reliable criteria for inferring a diagnostic label have to be sought, then the label should not have been brought into existence. And, even if a committee claims to have found reliable diagnostic criteria for a particular concept (as happens in the construction of the DSM), this claim can be disregarded, not because it is false, although experience tells us that it usually is, but because it is irrelevant to the crucial issue of validity. To claim to have found diagnostic criteria for an already existing concept is to imply that the concept's validity has already been established, otherwise how is its existence justified? But this cannot possibly be the case, because if it were, the committees would have no need to search for reliable diagnostic criteria.

To have to look for reliable diagnostic criteria for particular concepts or diagnostic labels, as so often happens in psychiatry, is therefore a reversal, some might say a travesty, of the usual scientific procedures for developing concepts. And it is because it is a travesty that we have such consistent reports of how very heterogeneous are the people who are grouped under the same category, indeed to the point where some people may have virtually nothing in common with others given the same diagnosis (see, e.g. Roth *et al.*, 1972; Weiner, 1989). It is for the same reason that research that tries to identify the underlying processes which account for the supposed surface pattern has been so unsuccessful and has consistently produced such inconsistent results. After all, you can't expect researchers, however well funded, to identify the processes which hold together a non-existent pattern.

The question arises then, of why and how psychiatric diagnosis has become so powerful, why its relationship to science should be so misrepresented. Obviously there is no one answer to this question, but four possible answers will be considered here. The first is that we seriously underestimate the difficulty of the process of developing the concepts that become diagnostic labels. There is a good deal of evidence that humans are very poor at many aspects of pattern recognition but that this does not stop us claiming to have seen relationships amongst all sorts of behaviours and characteristics (Kahneman *et al.*, 1982). One result of this is that we are over-accepting of psychiatry's claims about patterns of 'symptoms' which are said to justify diagnostic labels and do not subject them to the critical scrutiny they deserve. A second reason for the power of psychiatric diagnosis is that the knowledge needed to evaluate the diagnostic process in psychiatry is not easily available. It is therefore very difficult for ordinary people to know, to comment on or to challenge what is going on. This situation is not helped by psychiatry's spurious emphasis on reliability which gives the impression that important issues are being taken care of and that we need not enquire further.

Third, the existence of psychiatric diagnosis helps to allow apparently humane forms of social regulation under the authority of science. This means that challenging the scientific basis of psychiatric diagnosis is socially threatening because we then have to ask very searching questions about how to respond to psychological distress or to bizarre behaviour; about its relationship to social circumstances and to social structure, as well as questions about the apparent humanity of coercive psychiatry. It may be that both professionally and culturally we are willing to tolerate far lower standards of scrutiny of psychiatric diagnosis than we would of medical diagnosis because to do otherwise means facing these very difficult issues.

The fourth factor which maintains the power of psychiatric diagnosis is perhaps the most powerful of all. The diagnostic process involves a set of unarticulated assumptions about how we should think about people's behaviour, their experience and their distress. The DSM's claims to be atheoretical are entirely false; what makes them plausible is that the major theoretical assumption on which the DSM is based – that disturbing behaviour and experience should be thought of as if it were the equivalent of medical conditions such as rashes, fevers or cancerous tumours – is so pervasive in Western culture, so much part of our framework of thought, that we have ceased to see it *as* an assumption and instead treat it as a natural and immutable fact. Yet there is no evidence that this is a useful way to think about most behaviour and some very good evidence that it is not (e.g. Caplan, 1989; Johnstone, 1989; Weiner, 1989; Boyle, 1990). But so pervasive is this assumption that trying to develop a diagnostic system for psychological distress seems like the right thing to do, because that is, after all, the way medical conditions are recognized. Not only that, but since we already 'know' that mental disorders exist, then it seems reasonable to claim to have discovered particular types of disorder. And if the diagnostic system seems often to run into difficulties, if it cannot meet even the most basic requirement of reliable diagnostic criteria, then, we say, this is probably because these things take time, they are complex. What as a society we don't say, but is nearer the truth, is that the diagnostic enterprise is doomed always to run into problems because it is based on false premises.

Taken together, these factors help account for what I believe is the formidable power of psychiatric diagnosis. The juridical power of diagnosis is based on a false assumption of specialist knowledge which itself has created the impression that there exist 'out there' people suffering from naturally occurring mental disorders, only recognizable through a diagnostic process. This assumption of knowledge is in turn reinforced by the important social functions served by the diagnostic system. Each of these areas has to be confronted if we are to develop constructive alternatives to psychiatric diagnosis.

REFERENCES

American Psychiatric Association (1994) *Diagnostic and Statistical Manual of Mental Disorders,* 4th edn. Washington, DC: American Psychiatric Association.

Bean, P. (1980) *Compulsory Admissions to Mental Hospitals.* Chichester: Wiley.

Bentall, R.P. (1990) The Syndromes and Symptoms of Psychosis: Or why you can't play twenty questions with the concept of schizophrenia and hope to win. In: R.P. Bentall (ed.), *Reconstructing Schizophrenia.* London: Routledge.

Boyle, M. (1996) The fallacy of diagnosis. *Changes,* **14**: 5–13.

Boyle, M. (1990) *Schizophrenia: A Scientific Delusion?* London: Routledge.

Caplan, P.J. (1989) *Women's Masochism: The Myth Destroyed.* London: Mandarin.

Foucault, M. (1980) *Power/Knowledge. Selected Interviews and Other Writings, 1972–1977* (C. Gordon, ed.). Hemel Hempstead: Harvester Wheatsheaf.

Foucault, M. (1979) *A History of Sexuality,* vol. 1: *An Introduction.* London: Allen Lane.

Kirk, S.A. and Kutchins, H. (1992) *The Selling of DSM: the Rhetoric of Science in Psychiatry.* Hawthorne, NY: Walter deGruyter.

Johnstone, L. (1989) *Users and Abusers of Psychiatry.* London: Routledge.

Kahneman, D., Slovac, P. and Tversky, A. (1982) *Judgement under Uncertainty: Heuristics and Biases.* Cambridge: Cambridge University Press.

Roth, M., Gurney, C., Garside, R.F. and Kerr, T.A. (1972) Studies in the classification of affective disorders: the relationship between anxiety states and depressive illnesses. *British Journal of Psychiatry,* **121**: 147–161.

Sarbin, T.R. (1996) On the futility of psychiatric diagnostic manuals and the return of personal agency. Invited address to the 76th convention of the Western Psychological Association, San Jose, California, April.

Sawicki, J. (1991) *Disciplining Foucault: Feminism, Power and the Body.* London: Routledge.

Weiner, M. (1989) Psychopathology re-considered: depressions interpreted as psychosocial transactions. *Clinical Psychology Review,* **9**: 295–321.

Wing, J.K. (1988) Abandoning what? *British Journal of Clinical Psychology,* **27**: 325–328.

Suman Fernando

by Chris Stevenson

Suman Fernando is one of the most respected commentators in the UK on issues concerning the influences of race and culture in psychiatry. His interest has never been simply to comment, to be a wise yet distant figure in an increasingly volatile landscape. His work has traversed the whole psychiatric spectrum, from epidemiology to therapy, and he has also dedicated much of his time to supporting the development of meaningful community alternatives to mainstream psychiatry, and to organized citizen advocacy on behalf of people with mental health problems.

Suman Fernando was the ideal choice to address the increasingly complex issues surrounding race and culture in psychiatry. After a long and distinguished career he maintains his clinical position in the field, through his position as Honorary Consultant Psychiatrist at Chase Farm Hospital in Enfield, Middlesex. He is also a Senior Lecturer in Mental Health at the Tizard Centre at the University of Kent, Canterbury.

Suman is a member of the Council of Management of MIND, the national association for the promotion of mental health in the UK, which was founded at the end of the 1940s and which now commands the strongest voice, outside of Government, on mental health issues. He is also Chairperson of *Nafsiyat* Intercultural Therapy Centre and a member of various management committees of organizations dedicated to offering counselling services in the London area.

Suman's address to the conference reflected much of the man himself, as well as the standing of his thesis. He presented his arguments in a careful and reflective manner, indicative of a man who continues to ponder over the significance of the race and culture 'cards' and who is still seeking clarification of their exact meaning, in an increasingly multicultural Britain.

6

Imperialism, racism and psychiatry

Suman Fernando

In the early part of this century, the 'father' of psychiatry and the originator, to a large extent, of the German–British school of biological psychiatry, Kraepelin (1913), observed that guilt was not seen in Javanese people who became depressed – the Javanese, he said, were 'a psychically underdeveloped population' akin to 'immature European youth' (Kraepelin, 1921). This constellation of concepts epitomizes my own title here, 'Imperialism, racism and psychiatry'.

Throughout the first half of this century, the apparent rarity of depression among African-Americans and Africans was attributed to their 'irresponsible' and 'unthinking' nature (Green, 1914) or the 'absence of a sense of responsibility' (Carothers, 1953) in their character. In the 1920s, Carl Jung postulated that the 'Negro' 'has probably a whole historical layer less' in the brain (compared of course to white people) (Thomas and Sillen, 1972). Jung's layers referred to psychological development, analogous to anatomical layers of the cerebral cortex of the brain and his ideas could well have been influenced by numerous reports throughout the previous forty years that black people had smaller brains compared to white people (e.g. Bean, 1906). The first serious attempt to describe the psychiatry of black people (using 'black' in a broad sense) was in a textbook on adolescence by Stanley Hall (1904), where the psychology of Asians, Chinese, Africans and Indigenous Americans was described in a chapter headed 'Adolescent Races'. Indeed the idea that brown, yellow, black and red people are undeveloped white people ('akin to immature European youth' as Kraepelin put it) has had a strong influence on psychiatry and psychology throughout this century and has survived – some might say stabilized – into modern thinking.

One example is the continuation of discussions about IQ (i.e. Jensen, 1969; Eysenck, 1971; Rushton, 1990; Murray and Herrnstein, 1994; Brand,

1996). Another is the theory on emotional differentiation postulated by Julian Leff (1973), who analysed observations across the world made by psychiatrists trained in Western psychiatry to conclude that people from industrially underdeveloped countries and black Americans (the politically 'black') have a 'less developed' ability to differentiate emotions when compared with Europeans and white Americans. This 'evolutionary theory' (as Leff calls it) claims to explain why black people do not fall easily into the psychiatric categories – it is because they are underdeveloped in the ability to differentiate emotions; once the level of differentiation evolves to that of white people, there would be no problem.

Underdevelopment or the small brain thesis is not the only image of black people that informs clinical work and research within psychiatry and psychology. Before the last European war, Carl Jung (1930), on visiting the United States and observing what he called the 'striking peculiarities' of white Americans, postulated a psychological danger to white people from living too close to black people, i.e. his theory of 'racial infection':

> Now what is so contagious than to live side by side with a rather primitive people? Go to Africa and see what happened. When the effect is so very obvious that you stumble over it, then you call it 'going black' . . . The inferior man exercises a tremendous pull upon civilized beings who are forced to live with him, because it fascinates the inferior layers of our psyche, which has lived through untold ages of similar conditions. (1930: p. 195)

In analysing some of Jung's theories, Dalal (1988), a psychotherapist, believes that Jung's model for the mind of the infant was very similar in many ways to that for (what he called) 'primitive' humans. And, to Jung, blacks symbolized the primitive in himself. Perhaps here lies one source of the popular image that has developed (and affects psychiatry and psychology), the image of the dangers inherent in black people. The idea is that these dangers lurk in white people too but are kept well under control by higher layers of the mind, a control that the black person is not really capable of exerting to the same extent. This analysis is essentially similar to the scapegoating process, the projection on to 'the other' of all that one dislikes or fears in oneself, except that here, through psychiatry and therapy, efforts are made to control these dangerous feelings and behaviours – usually through medication or locking up. Frantz Fanon (1952: p. 121) wrote:

> In Europe, the black man is the symbol of Evil . . . In the remotest depths of the European unconscious an inordinately black hollow has been made in

which the most immoral impulses, the most shameful desires lie dormant. ... When European civilization came into contact with the black world, with those savage peoples, everyone agreed: those Negroes were the principle of evil. ... In the collective unconscious of *homo occidentalis* the Negro – or, if one prefers, the colour black – symbolizes evil, sin, wretchedness, death, war, famine.

As we all know, the events that took place in Europe during the 1930s, especially the Jewish holocaust in Germany, were deeply shocking to most Western Europeans and Americans (even it seems to Jung) and resulted in a revulsion against racist thinking with declarations by UNESCO denying the scientific validity of 'race' as a concept. However, it was perhaps significant that when WHO called on a specialist to write a monograph on African psychiatry, what should emerge but a report by J.C. Carothers, then the superintendent of a mental hospital in the British colony of Kenya, entitled *The African Mind in Health and Disease* (Carothers, 1953) in which, after repeating observation such as the lack of depression among Africans etc., Carothers concluded that the African mind resembled that of a 'leucotomized European', thus reviving the model of mental underdevelopment. And as I have already pointed out this ideology persists into the present.

The contention that psychiatry is basically and fundamentally racist, and cannot but continue to be racist as long as the profession fails to address this fact, is a view that I have developed in my book *Race and Culture in Psychiatry* (Fernando, 1988). Many people here would be familiar with the way psychiatry exerts power through its influence on the allocation of resources (e.g. as a gate-keeper to various types of help), its alienist function (its influence on decisions of society on who should be excluded from society and should not), and so on. At a personal level, psychiatry exerts power by its diagnostic procedure and the imposition of medication and other therapies to suppress, or at least interfere with, people's ideas, beliefs and feelings – and indeed even to alter family relationships. The power derives from insisting on psychiatric judgements and the results of psychological tests as *facts* or, at least *objective findings*; in other words, psychiatry through its so-called 'mental state examination':

1 Identifies 'pathology' which has to be suppressed, if not eradicated, *in the interests of the patient* (thus maintaining its patient-centred humane approach).
2 Identifies behaviours which have to be controlled or prevented from affecting the public, *in the interests of society* (referring to its responsibility to the community).
3 Acts to put things right.

When these judgements are integrated with racist perceptions of people, ideas, cultures and families, psychiatric power is combined with racism and race power manifested through psychiatry. How this is seen in ordinary practice is something I shall introduce, but first, where does all this come from?

HISTORY OF RACISM IN PSYCHIATRY

If we take a historical perspective it is not surprising that psychiatry is racist. After all, the disciplines of psychiatry and psychology developed together at a time when the powerful myths of racism were being refined and integrated into European culture, and it would have been very surprising if psychiatry had *not* developed a racist ideology. Psychiatry and psychology developed at the time when race thinking was the norm, even more strongly than it is now; when 'scientific racism' was being promoted as established knowledge; and when Social Darwinism placed different races at different levels on the ladder of evolution. Naturally, the culture of psychiatry included within it an ideology that saw anything to do with white people as superior to matters concerning black, brown, red and yellow people, so-called.

In the nineteenth century, psychiatrists in the US argued for the retention of slavery, quoting statistics allegedly showing that mental illness was more often reported among freed slaves compared to those who were still in slavery (Thomas and Sillen, 1972). When John Langdon Down (1866) surveyed so-called 'idiots' and 'imbeciles' resident in institutions around London, he identified them as 'racial throwbacks' to Ethiopian, Malay and Mongolian racial types – mostly, he said, they were 'Mongols'. And so it went on. And still carries on. The ideology of racism remains the same although the language changes. As Paul Gilroy (1987, 1993) writes, British racism in the 1990s 'frequently operates without any overt reference to "race" itself or the biological notions of difference which still give the term its common-sense meaning.' 'Culture', as an immutable, fixed property of social groups, has become confounded with 'race', and racism is articulated in cultural terms. Furthermore, racism is a major part of the ideology underlying the current discourse about nationality and belonging – about being 'British' or 'European'. In the words of the title of Gilroy's book, *There Ain't No Black in the Union Jack* (Gilroy, 1987). Nor it would seem in the blue flag with the circle of white stars (the flag of the European Community) or for that matter in the Stars and Stripes.

The exclusion of black people from a British identity comes through in day to day dealings in mental health care. For example, in examining the case notes of a black patient recently (on 26.2.96 of an entry made on

14.9.95), I noted that the key worker in evaluating 'Problems relating to culture (ethnicity)' stated:

> J-- is very conscious of her black identity though adamant that this is her country rather than Jamaica. She certainly considers that her Section 41 has not been lifted because she is black and that she is discriminated against because she is mentally ill and a woman.

IMPERIALISM

What we call imperialism is generally thought of as European power, to a large extent British power, which, from a European base (as it were) reached out and subjugated not just people but also cultures, languages etc. However, as McClintock (1995) puts it, 'imperial power emerged from a constellation of processes, taking haphazard shape from myriad encounters with alternative forms of authority, knowledge and power'. Clearly the underlying theme of imperialism has always been control and domination and imperialism has been backed by both personal and institutional violence. Yet, various policies and agendas were evident within imperialism, sometimes contradicting one another, some apparently humane, others barbaric. I have not the knowledge, time or ability to give you a comprehensive account of the ways in which imperial power was exercised. For present purposes, I have selected four of (what I have identified as) the tools used by imperialism, in order to discuss how they may apply today. I know that today we are supposed to be in a *post*-colonial era. I personally find it difficult to see how we can be *'post'* colonial if we take a global rather than eurocentric view. (Is colonialism 'post' in Palestine? In East Timor? In Tibet? In The Malvinas (Falklands)? In South Africa?) I cannot really see that there has been a clear cut-off from the colonial era, except perhaps in the minds of scholars of European literature. Imperialism has shifted, the players have changed a little, but the basic agenda remains the same.

1 Double standards

By double standards I essentially mean that ideas of justice and fair play applicable in the home country were not deemed suitable for colonial people. For example, even while Britain pursued slavery abroad, slavery was always illegal in Britain itself, leading to some well known legal cases involving runaway slaves; the imposition of the opium trade against the laws of China was pursued at a time when opium smoking was prohibited by law in England.

2 Industrial and cultural suppression

Undermining of local industries whenever these may compete with those of the home country was usually a policy instituted very early on after occupation. For example, paper making, textile, copper, brass and glass industries in India were all suppressed in the early 1800s. Imperial policy decreed that the colonies produced raw materials for British industry to create consumer goods for sale to the colonies. Even in the field of healing, literature and other cultural activities, the same policy applied. British medicine was imposed (and of course psychiatry went with that) while indigenous healing systems were suppressed often by law and always by underdevelopment.

3 Demonization

Right from the start of European domination, native healers were dubbed 'black magicians', or 'witch doctors' alluding to European traditions of abuse of the Middle Ages. As Bernal (1987) has shown in *Black Athena*, history itself was fundamentally distorted in the nineteenth century to deny the Afro-Asiatic roots of Greek culture: Chinese were demonized as opium addicts after Britain and France forced China to accept opium on a massive scale; Egyptian culture was separated off from African culture, black Africa demonized and Egypt white-washed. But most importantly for us today, a host of stereotypes, myths and imaginary stories were and are constructed and embedded in what we assume to be knowledge – often passed off as 'scientific' knowledge (via disciplines such as anthropology, psychology and psychiatry) – and embedded in 'common-sense', the common assumptions of ordinary people, not just among Western nations but much more generally. The images that play such a large part in perpetuating racism in psychiatry and psychology centre around dangerousness, passivity, lack of intelligence and, as I have mentioned earlier, the themes of under-development and demonization.

4 Divide and rule

Finally, the divide and rule strategy used and perpetuated division among conquered people, enticing favoured individuals and groups of people to participate in exercising imperial power.

MODERN IMPERIALISM

The era of the overseas empire in the old-fashioned sense has given way to – or more correctly been replaced by – neo-colonialism and economic domination, and now the new world order is directed by white America with British support. I shall not try to deal with the world scene but stay with our local scene – the British experience with a slight excursion into British activity overseas.

With the decline of direct power over colonies since the last European war, the empire has, as it were, come home to Britain. Since the 1950s we saw a reversal of what had happened for several centuries before that. Instead of Europeans moving out settling in other continents, people from Asia and Africa have been moving to Europe. This has of course now been stopped for, unlike in the earlier migration, the power positions do not favour migrants. As Stuart Hall and others pointed out in the 1970s, this migration of black people was recognized by British society as a threat and the control of black people became a political aim, although never actually voiced explicitly (Hall *et al.*, 1978). This control is no longer at arm's length (in far-flung colonies) but right here in Britain itself, in, as it were, internal colonies. The tools used clearly need modification or changing.

Democratic Britain could not have two sets of laws, one for black and one for white – at least not openly (although I believe that something very much like this, the foreigners laws, has emerged in Germany for the control of black people there). Britain could not restrict black people from using the educational services or establishing businesses – at least not officially. And this is where psychiatry comes into play.

In the 1960s a strong movement grew up protesting at the so-called 'abuse of psychiatry' in the old Soviet Union. In short, some political dissidents were being sent to secure hospitals having been diagnosed as schizophrenic because of their bizarre behaviour, delusional and grandiose ideas, etc. One thinks of a similar situation in the time of slavery in the United States when some runaway black slaves were diagnosed as suffering from drapetomania (mania for running away). Coming back to the Soviet Union, Foucault (1988) has pointed out that during Stalinist times, psychiatry had a very low profile. It was with liberalization under Kruschev that so-called abuse of psychiatry occurred. Actually it was not really 'abuse' as the 'use' of psychiatry for control and domination. It is likely that many of the diagnoses made were perfectly respectable within the psychiatric medical model. The people who were sent to hospital were indeed showing bizarre behaviour, they were irrational and quite unrealistic, they did have fantasies which any reasonable psychiatrist within the Soviet system would have interpreted as delusional.

In Britain today excessive numbers of black people are being diagnosed as 'schizophrenic' and being sent to secure hospitals and units.

In a context of racism where the control of black populations is clearly on the political agenda, the analogy with the Soviet Union is obvious. Psychiatrization has become a tool of imperialism. Of course it is not straightforward and psychiatry works through processes such as stereotyping on the basis of the sort of images and myths I have already discussed. For example, the 'big, black and dangerous' image was identified as an important factor in determining diagnosis and seclusion, meaning solitary confinement, in the inquiry into the deaths of black people in Broadmoor Secure Hospital (Special Hospitals Service Authority, 1993). Also, more general issues such as the association of both blackness and schizophrenia with violence, the medicalization of social problems allied to the power of the pharmaceutical firms peddling high-dose medication as a cure for all such 'illness' etc., all these are involved. But clearly, psychiatry is now one of the tools of imperialism for internal colonialism. This is not to say that all psychiatrists are personally racist. Just as some Soviet psychiatrists in the 1960s may have been KGB agents, some psychiatrists may well be prejudiced. However, it is the working of the psychiatric system that I am alluding to as racist. The trouble is that because of its very nature, its lack of much objectivity, its dependence on common-sense and poor validity of criteria used in diagnosis, psychiatry has always been – and as far as I can see always will be – open to permeation by social and political forces and so easily used to promote whatever power is dominant in society.

I said earlier that Britain cannot have different sets of laws and differential access to education based on race. This is of course so at an official level, but unofficially, the situation is that the legal system *does* operate differentially and barriers to advancement through education and economic progress are determined in part by race. I shall give two examples.

In commenting on recent cases of racially motivated murders, the *Observer* newspaper (28.4.96), in an editorial, contrasted the way the police and the Crown Prosecution Service handled the murder case of Stephen Lawrence (a black youngster murdered in April 1993) with that of Richard Everitt (a white youngster murdered in August 1994). Within a few hours of the killing of Stephen Lawrence, the local police had numerous approaches from the public, in which those allegedly responsible were named: but no arrests were made for more than a fortnight by which time vital evidence had disappeared. This time lapse directly caused the failure of the case, because it allowed time for the identification witness to pick up the gossip from the street. This, the defence argued successfully, meant the witness's identification might be 'contaminated'. In contrast, said the editorial, following Richard Everitt's equally brutal murder, police 'charged into the local Asian centre and picked up no fewer than 300 Asian youths'. The man charged was jailed on the grounds of 'joint enterprise' even though it was acknowledged that he did not wield the knife that killed Richard Everitt.

The second example is from the field of education. In 1986, after information from researchers at St George's Hospital Medical School, the Commission for Racial Equality (1988) uncovered the existence of an unofficial but extremely effective method by which racial designation was used to exclude differentially applicants for medical education. And these instances are clearly just the tips of several icebergs of institution-alized racism that exists in spite of 'equality before the law'.

I have argued so far, I think, that racist imperialism finds its implementation through psychiatry in the local British scene through the diagnosis of schizophrenia, compulsory treatment etc. What happens at an international level is perhaps rather different. As far as we know, the diagnosis of schizophrenia is not related to racial difference in ex-colonial countries, such as Jamaica. There may be many reasons for this and I cannot go into this here. What does happen, I think, at a global level is that imperialism is involved in some, at least, of the procedures and policies, concerning mental health through something very much like the third set of tools in my new list – industrial and cultural suppression.

The example I have is the International Pilot Study of Schizophrenia of the WHO (World Health Organization, 1973, 1979) – the IPSS. This large project began in 1966 using people presenting at hospitals in nine centres in Denmark, India, Columbia, Nigeria, the United Kingdom, the USSR, Czechoslovakia, Taiwan and USA. The diagnosis was based on a combination of standardized schedules on history, social status and, most importantly, the Present State Examination (PSE). This last crucial instrument is (to quote its founder) 'a special technique of interviewing patients, ... which is simply a standardized form of the psychiatric diagnostic interview ordinarily used in Western Europe, based on a detailed glossary of differential definition of symptoms' (Wing, 1978). What is so remarkable for an expensive study is that no attempt was made to establish the validity of the measuring tools – no attempt to see whether a 'diagnosis' based on such tools had any meaning or usefulness as 'illness' in the countries concerned. This mistake in research method-ology has been dubbed 'category fallacy' by Kleinman (1977), but the WHO continues to use a similar approach in the successor to the IPSS, the Determinants of Outcomes of Severe Mental Disorder (DOSMD) (Jablensky *et al.*, 1992). Cultural arrogance or is it racist imperialism? Is there a difference?

Incidentally, a significant finding of this study (Leff *et al.*, 1992) is that people diagnosed as 'schizophrenic' in the industrially under-developed parts of the world (where traditional Western treatments and follow-up is minimal) have (in medical terms) a better prognosis than those in industrially developed countries (where such treatments are usually applied). In other words the diagnosis does not appear to predict the usefulness of traditional Western treatment to say the least – that is, if the diagnosis is a valid one for identifying a particular condition.

I do not wish to get into the broader issue of the validity of schizophrenia as 'illness' anyway, but the point that I am making here is that imposing Western models of illness irrespective of what the natives think represents the imperialism of psychiatry. As with other aspects of imperial policy, there are inherent economic advantages in ensuring that the manufacturing base for psychiatry remains in the home country, after all the drug firms are here, the centres of excellence are here, the potential governors who would go out to train the natives are here. Clearly, the overall agenda of international imperialism has not changed very much but, as a sort of superficial liberalization has taken place with the dismantling of colonies, psychiatry has come into play.

To complete the picture of modern imperialism, 'demonization' continues to be used but in a different form. For example, a subtle criminalization of social problems affect black people in Britain dispro-portionately. As for 'divide-and-rule' we can see this (for example) in the way that prestigious institutes that govern psychiatry adopt and promote black individuals who play the imperial game while 'cooling out' those who do not.

So perhaps the original tools of imperialism have been modified to suit the times.

CONCLUSIONS

Early psychiatrists were called 'Alienists', people responsible for deter-mining who was 'alien' to society and who was not. And designating human problems in terms of 'illness' or people requiring 'help' became very mixed up with social control of people. The original eugenic movement that justified, indeed promoted, the genocide in Germany (of Jews, Gypsies etc.) arose within clinical psychology (e.g. Francis Galton), supported by psychiatrists (e.g. Kraepelin in Germany) wishing to 'cleanse' society (the movement for mental hygiene). Today, the so-called violence initiatives in the United States involves psychiatrists and psychologists identifying children for treatment to prevent them becom-ing dangerous. And of course the everyday work of psychiatrists in compulsory detention and forced medication is a natural part of our social system codified in the Mental Health Act. *Racism is involved in both instances.*

In the 1960s we saw in Britain a shift in psychiatry towards liberalization and a sort of 'enlightenment' about mental health with understanding and care superseding control and management. There was even a tendency to loosen the medical model – at least in service provision – away from the so-called centres of excellence at any rate. The 1980s and 1990s, however, have seen a reversal of these trends for various reasons. Today, Kraepelinian psychiatry, with firm diagnostic categories and biological explanations, is again popular, now on both sides of the

Atlantic, and authoritarian psychiatric interventions are being promoted again as 'social psychiatry'. Assertive outreach has come to mean controlling interventions *in* the community, nearly always through medication. And racism is quite definitely involved, often couched in cultural terms.

In such a context, stereotypical assumptions about black people influence assessments that professionals make. The fact is that with racism involved, with a system such as psychiatry that exercises power through diagnosis, and with an inheritance through imperialism of damaging stereotypes that construct images of dangerousness, madness and alienness, the fact is that, just as some nineteenth century American psychiatrists saw run away slaves as *drapetomanic*, it is not difficult for *us* to see angry, undesirable, 'aliens' as '*schizophrenic*' or '*psychotic*' – and that is exactly what does happen and that is how racism operates, that is how imperialism operates, that is how psychiatry operates, not all the time of course and not for everyone but often enough. Of course when major tranquillizers are called on and feelings and behaviour are suppressed, a self-fulfilling prophecy appears to confirm 'clinical acumen' in diagnosis – appears to justify the use of power.

SUMMARY

I have tried to trace here the interplay between imperialism, psychiatry and racism. As the direct application of imperialism has changed under new forces (for example, so-called de-colonization), psychiatry has come into play as an imperial force carrying (as imperialism always did) racism within it. In other words, the imperialism carried over from slavery and colonialism is now being manifested through psychiatry – both in the exercise of racist power over black people within Britain and through the imposition of psychiatric models overseas. The over-diagnosis of black people as schizophrenic and their confinement as detained patients or over-medicated zombies in the community is one result. Overseas, the imposition of Western psychiatric categories ensures the dominance of Western ideas and accrues economic advantages. The tools of modern imperialism remain the same or similar to those used in the past.

It is difficult to see how this continuation of the colonial era can be stopped. Concentrating on reforming psychiatry alone is not the answer since much wider issues are involved. However, examining the psychiatric system, the power of the system, its racism, its *real* function in society could be a start or at least a *part* of the struggle for black people in contending with imperialism, confronting racism and incidentally surviving psychiatry.

REFERENCES

Bean, R.B. (1906) Some racial peculiarities of the Negro brain. *American Journal of Anatomy*, **5**: 353–415.

Bernal, M. (1987) Black Athena. *The Afroasiatic Roots of Classical Civilization*, vol. 1. London: Free Association.

Brand, C. (1996) *The g Factor. General Intelligence and its Implications.* Chichester: Wiley.

Carothers, J.C. (1953) *The African Mind in Health and Disease. A Study in Ethnopsychiatry.* WHO Monograph Series No. 17. Geneva: World Health Organization.

Commission for Racial Equality (1988) *Medical School Admission. Report of a Formal Investigation into St George's Hospital Medical School.* London: CRE.

Dalal, F. (1988) The racism of Jung. *Race and Class*, **29**: 1–22.

Down, J.L.M. (1866) Observations on an ethnic classification of idiots. *Lectures and Reports from the London Hospital for 1866*, reprinted in C. Thompson (ed.) (1987) *The Origins of Modern Psychiatry.* Chichester: Wiley, pp. 15–18.

Eysenck, H.J. (1971) *Race, Intelligence and Education.* London: Temple Smith.

Fanon, F. (1952) *Peau Noire, Masques blancs.* (Transl. C. L. Markham). Paris: Editions de Seuil.

Fernando, S. (1988) *Race and Culture in Psychiatry.* London: Croom Helm. Reprinted as paperback (1989), London: Routledge.

Fernando, S., Ndegwa, D. and Wilson, M. (1998) *Forensic Psychiatry, Race and Culture.* London: Routledge.

Foucault, M. (1988) *Politics, Philosophy, Culture: Interviews and other writings. 1977–84.* Edited by L. D. Kritzman. New York: Routledge.

Gilroy, P. (1987) *There Ain't No Black in the Union Jack.* London: Routledge.

Gilroy, P. (1993) One nation under a groove. In: *Small Acts. Thoughts on the Politics of Black Cultures.* London: Serpent Tail, pp. 19–48.

Green, E.M. (1914) Psychoses among Negroes – a comparative study. *Journal of Nervous and Mental Disorder*, **41**: 697–708.

Hall, G.S. (1904) *Adolescence its Psychology and its Relations to Physiology, Anthropology, Sociology, Sex, Crime, Religion and Education*, vol. 2. New York: Appleton.

Hall, S., Critcher, C., Jefferson, T., Clarke, J. and Roberts, B. (1978) *Policing the Crisis: Mugging, the State, and Law and Order.* London: Macmillan.

Harrison, G., Owens, D., Holton, A., Neilson, D. and Boot, D. (1988) A prospective study of severe mental disorder in Afro-Caribbean patients. *Psychological Medicine*, **18**: 643–657.

Jablensky, A., Sartorius, N., Ernberg, G., Anker, M., Korten, A., Day, R. *et al.* (1992) Schizophrenia: manifestations, incidence and course in different cultures. A World Health Organization ten-country study. *Psychological Medicine Monograph Supplement*, **20**: 1–97.

Jensen, A.R. (1969) How much can we boost IQ and scholastic achievement? *Harvard Educational Review*, **39**: 1–123.

Jung, C.G. (1930) Your Negroid and Indian behaviour. *Forum*, **83**(4): 193–199.

Kleinman, A. (1977) Depression, somatization and the 'New Cross-Cultural Psychiatry'. *Social Science and Medicine*, **11**: 3–10.

Kraepelin, E. (1913) *Manic Depressive Insanity and Paranoia* (translation of *Lehrbuch der Psychiatrie*, R. M. Barclay), 8th edn, vols 3 and 4. Edinburgh: Livingstone.

Kraepelin, E. (1921) *Manic Depressive Insanity and Paranoia* (trans. and edited R.M. Barclay and G.M. Robertson). Edinburgh: Livingstone.

Leff, J. (1973) Culture and the differentiation of emotional states. *British Journal of Psychiatry*, **123**: 299–306.

Leff, J., Sartorius, N., Jablensky, A. and Ernberg, G. (1992) The International Pilot Study of Schizophrenia: five year follow up findings. *Psychological Medicine*, **22**: 131–145.

McClintock, A. (1995) *Imperial Leather: Race, Gender and Sexuality in the Colonial Contest*. London: Routledge.

McGovern, D. and Cope, R. (1987) The compulsory detention of males of different ethnic groups, with special reference to offender patients. *British Journal of Psychiatry*, **150**: 505–512.

Murray, C. and Herrnstein, R. (1994) *The Bell Curve: Intelligence and Class Structure in American Life*. New York: Free Press.

Rushton, C. (1990) Race differences, r/K theory, and a reply to Flynn. *The Psychologist: Bulletin of the British Psychological Society*, **5**: 195–198.

Special Hospitals Service Authority (SHSA) (1993) *Report of the Committee of Inquiry into the Death in Broadmoor Hospital of Orville Blackwood and a Review of the Deaths of Two Other Afro-Caribbean Patients: 'Big, Black and Dangerous?'* (Chairman Professor H. Prins). SHSA, London.

Thomas, A. and Sillen, S. (1972) *Racism and Psychiatry*. New York: Brunner/ Mazel.

Wing, J.K. (1978) *Reasoning about Madness*. Oxford: Oxford University Press.

World Health Organization (1973) *Report of the International Pilot Study of Schizophrenia*, vol. 1. Geneva: WHO.

World Health Organization (1979) *Schizophrenia: an International Follow-up Study*. London: Wiley.

Introduction to Chapter 7

Marius Romme

by Chris Stevenson

Marius Romme is Professor in Social Psychiatry at the University of Maastricht, The Netherlands. This formal title does not convey the warmth of the man who it was my privilege to meet at the Longhirst Conference. I had no doubts that Romme, the clinician, would be able to engage in a humane and connected way with the voice hearers he works with.

There is a wealth of evidence to support my assessment. It takes a special kind of concern to have founded the Hearing Voices Network with which Romme has become synonymous. Functioning internationally, the network has offered a special kind of sanctuary to those living with a voice experience. An asylum from the asylum. Part of the uniqueness of the Hearing Voices movement has been the avoidance of professionally driven agendas for the network. Consequently, Romme has succeeded in providing a demedicalized account of the voice experience. He has written a book, *Accepting Voices* (published in 1993 by MIND), which has been translated into six languages, for people who know the experience of hearing voices, as well as texts for psychiatric professionals.

Marius Romme's ability to blur the boundary between the normal and abnormal is the most striking aspect of his work. People who hear voices do not always fall foul of psychiatric systems, can lead lives indistinguishable from non-voice hearers. His work with Sondra Escher has challenged the preoccupation in psychiatry with individual psychopathology. Now there is room for understanding voice experiences as part of the human repertoire, for appreciating that voices are not arbitrary, but carry significance in terms of the life story of the individual.

7

'Hearing voices': madness or communication?

Marius Romme

The authority of psychiatry is based on the existence of discrete illness entities and the knowledge of the psychiatric profession about their origin; their symptomatic expression; their course, outcome and treatment.

The problem presented by such a basis for professional authority in relation to psychotic illnesses, is that all these aspects of the supposed illness entities lack scientific validity and therefore are no more than beliefs. These views were formulated a century ago by Kraepelin who tried to make a diagnostic system out of the different behaviour patterns of patients he observed in clinical practice. At that time it was an advance to include psychiatric disorders within the ambit of healthcare and out of the guilt-burdened moralistic approach. However, nowadays these attitudes have become counterproductive and a drawback in the patients' development and have been proved to be not scientifically valid.

The main issues of the Kraepelinian conceptualization are:

1 Psychotic symptoms can be divided into small numbers of discrete clusters representing different illnesses.
2 The psychotic symptoms a person shows result from one of these different illnesses.
3 Psychotic symptoms are not understandable and do not reflect patients' personalities and experiences.
4 The different psychotic illnesses are stress provoked but based on vulnerabilities caused by specific brain disorders.

Despite the above, all psychiatrists agree, from their own observations, that schizophrenia, as an example of these psychotic illnesses, has no consistent pattern of symptoms, it has no particular known cause, and does not respond in any predictable way to any known treatment.

However Kraepelinian concepts are still the basis of mainstream psychiatric practice. It is as if psychiatry is still proud of that formulation, proud that they did not have to change the concept and were able to defend it a for a hundred years, despite it still needing scientific validity, and still not knowing the causes. They still don't listen to what people who experience these illnesses have to tell us about those experiences and therefore still don't have an alternative for their illness-entity idea. Mary Boyle has explained what is lacking on the level of scientific validity of the concept (see Chapter 5) and Alec Jenner (see Chapter 9) has indicated why the causal influence of the so-called dopamine neurotransmission hypothesis seems to be wrong when the effect of a new more powerful antipsychotic drug, clozapine, works differently. I want to discuss how listening to the people who have experienced psychotic disorder might lead to an alternative concept for those disorders which are more in tune with the concepts around neurotic disorders.

This alternative is an alternative within healthcare but emphasizes personalities and experiences, instead of excluding them.

My interest and that of my colleagues (Romme *et al.*, 1992) in the experience of 'hearing voices' began some years ago. One of my patients was a 30-year-old woman who had heard voices 'in her mind'. These voices gave her orders to forbid her to do certain things, dominating her completely and, as a result, she had been hospitalized several times and diagnosed as having schizophrenia. Neuroleptics had no effect on the voices, although they did reduce the anxiety provoked by them. However, the medication also reduced her mental alertness. In order to stay alert, she stopped taking medication over a long period of time, not staying long as an inpatient when she required to be hospitalized. Nevertheless, the voices isolated her more and more by forbidding her to do the things she always loved to do.

One year she began to talk about suicide and I felt that she had reached a turning point. The only positive topic in our communication was the theory she had developed about the phenomenon of the voices. This was based on a book written by the American psychologist Julian Jaynes (1976), *The Origin of Consciousness in the Breakdown of the Bicameral Mind*. It was reassuring for her to read the author's report of people hearing voices as a 'normal way of making decisions' until about 1300 BC. According to Jaynes, hearing voices has disappeared and been replaced by what we now call 'consciousness'.

I began to wonder if this woman could communicate effectively with other people who 'heard voices' and whether her theory would be accepted by other people who appeared to have similar experiences. I thought that this might have a positive effect on her sense of isolation and her suicidal tendencies. She and I began to plan together how she might share some of those experiences and also her views about what was happening. The end result was the establishment of our research and the development of the 'Hearing Voices Network'.

We have tried to listen to what people say about their experience, especially to those who hear voices. When you listen, you hear that they do not experience an illness *(per se)*, but that they have perceptions that frighten them, that puzzle them, disturb them in their daily actions or that sometimes give good advice and then capture their interest. It is mostly distress that brings people to a psychiatrist. What the voices say is very personal and differs from person to person.

WHAT WE LEARNT FROM VOICE HEARERS: THE DUTCH EXPERIENCE

The negative side

We learned that the most puzzling symptom – the voices – were present a long time before other symptoms developed. And when these people went to a psychiatrist they say that they usually did not get a satisfactory answer. They had developed an understanding themselves, one not based on our reality but on their experience, for example, feeling telepathically influenced, being followed, hearing ghosts, feeling energies etc. These explanations are called delusions within the traditional concept and seen as the result of the underlying illness, but they might also be interrelated to the perception of hearing voices, for instance as an explanation following a not otherwise comprehensible perception. The next step in the sequence of developing their reactive behaviour might contain coping strategies in order to adapt to their perceptions and be less hindered by them. This might entail not answering the phone in the evening; staying in bed to avoid doing what the voices say and in such a way avoiding expressing their aggression; or performing other rituals to keep control over their emotions. The voices also might disturb their orientation so they might avoid meeting many people, or they avoid visiting certain places etc. These are all kinds of behaviour that are then called the negative symptoms of schizophrenia within the traditional outlook.

This, however, might also indicate that symptoms are interrelated with each other and not only the result of an underlying illness. Other examples of this interrelation are: concentration disturbances and inadequate affect, which may both be the direct effect of being disturbed by a voice distracting one's attention and provoking emotions. Other symptoms, like socially inadequate conduct, might be the result of coping with the disturbing voices in an attempt to keep control, as in obsessive–compulsive neurosis.

This interrelation of symptoms which will be different in different persons, might point to an alternative explanation of the illness concept.

It was Ron Coleman (see Chapter 4) who made us realize that it might be possible that the sequence of the different symptoms in time indicates that one symptom might provoke the other symptoms. Looking at it this way might indicate that the coping difficulties experienced in response to the first most puzzling symptom, actually provokes the illness. Therefore it is not the illness that provokes the symptoms but the *symptom that provokes the illness.*

This alternative explanation however needs to be complemented by an appreciation of what might lie at the basis of that first symptom. In our research (Romme and Escher, 1989; Romme *et al.*, 1992) we found the basis for hearing voices is the person's personality and experiences.

Before I report on that relationship, I will explain why we went looking for such a relationship. This was due to the following positive aspects about hearing voices. Again we learned these by listening to the people who hear them.

The positive side

We learned for instance that you could hear voices and never become a psychiatric patient. We learned from others that what the voices said had a meaning for them, which they have learned to understand. We also learned that voices for some people have a signal function, indicating a daily stress difficult to overcome. Some others experienced that when they solved their problems they did not need the voices any more. Most importantly, we also learned that if a person who hears voices is able to give that voice his or her own voice to speak out in the outer world, then life becomes a challenge again. Instead of the person becoming a victim they became the owner, they could take their life into their own hands and break through the vicious circle of dependence on the voices and the authority of the voices. Because of what we were told we started a study focusing on this 'hearing voices' phenomenon.

THE STUDY

The study compared three groups of persons hearing voices, two patient groups and one non-patient group. In the two patient groups one group was diagnosed as having schizophrenia and one diagnosed as having a dissociative disorder. All the respondents were hearing voices with the characteristics of auditory hallucinations. That means hearing someone speaking without an observable source and experiencing the voice(s) as 'not me' but someone or something else.

To differentiate between the two patient groups, we used the CIDE = Composed International Diagnostic Interview (Robins *et al.*, 1988) and the DES = Dissociative Experience Scale (Putnam and Bernstein, 1986).

We recruited the respondents from a community mental health centre after an inventory of all the patients referred to this centre who were asked whether they did or did not hear voices. We selected, with these instruments, a group of 15 patients diagnosed as schizophrenic, a group of 15 patients diagnosed as having a dissociative disorder. The non-patients hearing voices were recruited through TV and print media.

We gathered information about the voices with a semi-structured interview containing the following items:

- Aspects of the experience itself.
- Characteristics of the voices heard.
- The circumstance present when hearing voices began.
- Triggers – now.
- Identity of the voices.
- Interpretations of the voices.
- Coping strategies.
- Social network – now.
- Experiences in childhood.

Our main points of interest and main results arose from the following questions:

1 Do the formal criteria of auditory hallucinations differ between the three groups, e.g. are the Schneiderian criteria specific for schizophrenia?
2 Is there a difference between the three groups in the influence of the voices on the person who hears them?
3 Are their differences in the involvement with the voices?
4 Are there differences in the relationship between the voices and the life history between the three groups? For instance does a dissociative disorder relate to a traumatic event and is this not the case in schizophrenia? And what about the non-patients?

Do the formal criteria differ between the three groups?

The formal criteria that are used in psychiatric epidemiological research like the WHO pilot study on schizophrenia are supposed to differentiate between so-called 'real' or 'pseudo' hallucinations. The real hallucinations were seen as symptoms relating to schizophrenia. The differentiations between the perception of the real and pseudo-hallucinations were considered to be:

1 The way the voice is heard by the ears or in the head.
2 The experience of the voice as 'not me' or 'possibly me'.

3 The ability of the person to communicate with the voice or not.
4 The way the voice speaks to the person in the third or second person.

No distinctive features emerged between the three groups on any of the measures mentioned above. In other words, psychiatric criteria were irrelevant in ascertaining who should be a patient. In all three groups voices are heard 'by the ears' as well as 'in the head'. Voices are experienced as not me in most cases of all groups. The possibility of communicating with the voices slightly differs between the dissociative disordered and the other two but in a controversial way because in psychiatry it is suggested that schizophrenia patients do not communicate with their voices. The last criterion also does not show the expected differences. Schizophrenics do not hear more third person voices than other groups and the other groups hear as much commenting voices as the schizophrenics do.

Does the influence of the voices differ between the three groups?

Here we found a rather important difference between the patient groups and the non-patient group due to the content of the voices and the beliefs about the voices.

The patient groups experience the voices as dominantly negative, while the non-patient group experience the voices as dominantly positive. Another difference is that the patient groups are afraid of the voices, which is not the case with the non-patient group. The third difference is that the patient groups are disturbed by the voices in the performance of their daily activities while this is much less the case in the non-patients. The two patient groups do not differ from each other, they both are afraid of the voices, are disturbed by them in the performance of their daily activities and experience the voices as predominantly negative or threatening.

The relationship between the life history experiences and the hearing voices experience

This is a more complicated issue. We differentiated the information about the life history into what happened at the time the voices began and what had happened during upbringing. This in itself is a rather normal psychiatric way of information-gathering with neurotic illness. So why not do it in psychotic illness?

In all three groups there is a differing but rather high coincidence between negatively experienced circumstances and the beginning of the voices. These were thought to be important by the patient in initiating the voices. These events, however, differ in the impact they had on the person's life history and also might be differently coped with. Like in all traumatic events, their influence on the life history differs between individuals. They might have a disrupting impact but that does not need to be the case. What we perceived in our study is that if a person is made powerless by the events or circumstances, he or she also is powerless towards the voices. Those who are not made powerless by the events also behave more defensibly towards the voices. A few examples might illustrate this interaction:

Example: a patient diagnosed as dissociative-disordered
As a girl of 9 years old she had been beaten so severely by her father that she was admitted to hospital because two vertebra had been damaged. Two hours after admission she heard voices for the first time. This girl recovered bodily completely and was placed at her grandmother's house, which was a comfortable and safe surrounding for her. So at first there was no negative consequence for her connected with the trauma. However, three years later her grandmother died and she was then admitted to a home. In this institution there was no more safety than in her father's house. Here, education and good behaviour were aggressively forced upon her, and she may have been more sensitive for that behaviour. She became too vulnerable to cope with the voices.

Example: a patient diagnosed as having schizophrenia
A 40-year-old man starts hearing voices a few days before he has to do an examination that is vital to keep his job and which he realizes that he will certainly fail because the requirements are too heavy for him. In his life history this trauma was a kind of repetition. He was vulnerable and could not cope because in his youth he had been belittled by his father and been thought stupid with the consequence that his brother was made the father's successor so that he had to look for a profession elsewhere, which now he was threatened with losing.

Example: a non-patient hearing voices
A 40-year-old woman starts hearing voices after the loss by death of three very important persons in her life – her husband, her father and her sister-in-law – all in a period of three months. She did not

become a patient. This was emotionally a trauma but it did not bring negative consequences to her life. She did not have to change her life neither financially nor had she to change housing or lose her children. Furthermore her history showed a youth and education in which she was very much stimulated and supported. She developed a stable identity and was not that vulnerable when she suffered the losses.

The great difference between patients and non-patients both hearing voices seems to be:

1 The different consequences a traumatic event around the beginning of the hearing voices has on one's life. In patients we see a more long-term negative impact than in non-patients.
2 The differences in positive or negative experience during life before the hearing voices happens. For example, how securely the person grew up or how insecure s/he became. Or how strong or defective the person's identity has become before arriving at the event which initiated the voices.

CONCLUSIONS

The symptom of 'auditory hallucination' lies on a continuum with normal functioning. It is not the *hearing of voices* that indicates psychopathology but the way a person copes with voices that creates psychopathology. It is not wrong to call defective coping with hearing voices psychotic but it is problematic that psychiatry looks at the phenomena in a different way compared with how neurotic problems are looked at.

Psychotic phenomena have a meaning in the person's life history and can be very well understood from the patient's personality and experiences. Persons who become patients can be helped in their coping. Although the life history cannot be changed the influence it still has can. This is not an easy job for the patient and there will be some people who will perceive this job as too threatening. The perception as well as the acceptance of certain feelings may not be possible.

This study taught us how psychiatry diagnoses can function as a handicap for the patients. The traditional diagnostic concept implies that the symptoms are coming from the illness, which makes the person powerless. This is not the case as the symptoms can be seen as a person's way of relating to his or her personality and experiences.

The relationship between the first symptom and the life history might indicate that vulnerability is not necessarily a biological vulnerability, but might well be built up during life in the interaction with others. The difference in vulnerability between patients and non-patients both hearing voices might indicate that the illness is not the cause of the symptom but that the symptom might cause illness.

REFERENCES

Jaynes, J. (1976) *The Origin of Consciousness in the Breakdown of the Bicameral Mind.* Boston: Houghton and Mifflin.

Putnam, F.W. and Bernstein, E.M. (1986) Development, reliability and validity of a dissociation scale. *Journal of Nervous and Mental Disease,* **174**: 727–35.

Robins, L.N., Wing, H.U. and Wittchen, E.A. (1988) The composite international diagnostic interview. *Archives of General Psychiatry,* **174**: 727–35.

Romme, M.A.J and Escher, A.D.M. (1989) Hearing voices. *Schizophrenia Bulletin* **15**(2): 209–216.

Romme, M.A.J., Honig, A., Noorthoorn, E.O. and Escher, A.D.M. (1992) Coping with hearing voices: an emancipator approach. *British Journal of Psychiatry,* **16**: 99–103.

Introduction to Chapter 8

Shulamit Ramon

by Chris Stevenson

Shulamit (Shula) Ramon has an unusual background in that she is trained as a social worker and clinical psychologist. She has worked as a senior lecturer at the London School of Economics, but currently holds a chair in Social Policy at Anglia Polytechnic University.

Shula has researched and published widely in the area of psychiatric community care, making valuable cross-national comparisons. Over the past few years, she has developed an increasing involvement with countries from the former Eastern bloc and has led the development of social work training in parts of the former Soviet Union. These international interests serve to reflect many of the deeply held convictions about the plight of both the mental health worker and the clientele whom they serve. In this chapter, Shula focuses her attention on many of the uncertainties – both philosophical, political and practical – which continue to influence the development of mental health services at home, as well as abroad.

Her special ability to ask searching questions about existing social policy underpins her formidable talent in debating. These qualities were much in evidence at the Longhirst Conference, where she was careful to integrate some of the thoughts she had brought with her to the conference, with the flow of the proceedings. In my view this reflected, at least in part, the organic nature of her thinking: trying constantly to find the mirror for her own philosophy.

If there is one quality which underpins this wide-ranging view of policy, politics and practice, it is the need to balance the rhetorical with the practical – especially where madness is invoked. Her expression of compassion was also evident at the conference, often in overtly empathic terms, for mental health workers, who might be as dispossessed as some of the people for whom they carried great responsibility, at least in the politicized eye of the service managers. How we confront the tensions of competing demands from the legislature and simple, human need, is a challenge which Shula accepts readily, as a careful reading of this chapter will show.

8

Living with ambiguity and ambivalence: mental health workers' perspective

Shulamit Ramon

I am starting from the assumption that if mental health professionals did not exist, we would need to re-invent them. They are essential for crisis work, long-term work, family work, reflective work with individual clients, prescribing and administering medication.

Ivan Illich and others have argued since the 1960s that professional activity is disabling (Illich, 1968) because it prevents people from sorting out their own problems on their own. While there is an element of truth in this argument, it is one which ignores the sociological fact that professions have arisen in a society stripped of a number of supportive networks which have existed in the past. Specifically relating this concept to mental distress, total reliance on professional approaches is undesirable in my view, while doing away with professional knowledge and support is likewise undesirable in terms of people's needs in a hostile world.

However, in this process of re-invention I would like to see created professionals who are genuinely engaged in partnership with clients, who look for and foster abilities in their clients and the relatives of the latter, who follow a psychological approach, and who are ready to give up their (largely controlling) power in this process. For me, professional knowledge is one perspective among a number of equally valid knowledge frameworks; professionals are one group of stakeholders among a number of stakeholders in the field of mental distress.

To be able to go about the re-invention it is useful to attempt to understand the issues, the ambiguities and ambivalences, which all mental health professionals live with.

This discussion will have two parts:

1 Focusing on issues which are typical of mental health work anywhere, including Britain.
2 Focusing on issues specific to the current British context.

GLOBAL ISSUES

Professionals in mental distress services are described as:

- weak, conservative and ineffectual because of the hegemony of manageralism and political interference in the Western world;
- all too powerful, yet ineffectual, because they are impervious to users' and relatives' needs, defying management attempts to tame them;
- ineffectual because the knowledge base is so underdeveloped;
- ineffectual and conservative because of the value base of these professions, especially that of medically related staff;
- effectual in some respects, but not in others, because of the enormity and complexity of the field and the tasks.

The acceptance of one of these statements or the other leads to different conclusions and directions as to what is wrong, what is right and what needs to be changed in relation to mental distress professions.

Before we turn to look at the implications of these statements, I would like to dwell a bit on the fact that *all four* can be held concurrently, though usually not by the same person/group, regardless of the wide gap among them, and the contrasting logic underlying them. This is possible not only because different stakeholders in psychiatry may have different perspectives on the subject matter, but also due to shifts in power given and taken from professionals, and the very nature of their authority.

It might be useful to begin by understanding a bit better the latter component. Beckman (1990) proposed that the root of this authority goes back to its Latin meaning, namely the explication of secretive texts and dogmas to laymen by authorized experts. It is an authority for action, belief, valuation and being given to professionals by others who voluntarily comply with the instructions provided by professionals (1990: 126). Usually this authority is given by society at large, rather than by the individuals most affected by it, because the latter are not perceived as a credible authority source. When there is also a *formal* obligation to follow authority this is likely to imply lack of voluntary acceptance of its credibility (e.g. compulsory admission).

Weber has proposed what has become a classical typology of authority: traditional, institutional, legal, rational-neutral, charismatic and personal.

Curiously, professional authority is a mixture of the rational-neutral and the charismatic types of authority. Similarly it lies between the institutional and the personal. It also relies on the assumed personal incompetence of the others.

According to the *Shorter Oxford Dictionary*, the earliest meaning of 'professed' was: 'that has taken the vows of a religious order'. By 1675, the secular meaning attached implied:

> that professes to be duly qualified: professional ... the occupation which one professes to be skilled in and to follow ... a vocation in which professed knowledge of some branch of learning is used in its application to the affairs of others, or in the practice of an art based upon it. Applied specifically to the three learned professions of divinity, law and medicine; also the military profession.

The *vocational* element is important, because it sets these professions apart from occupations in which work is aimed at enabling one to earn her/his living first, to offer any other satisfactions second; and to provide a service focused on meeting people's need third, if at all. A vocation implies a mission and a commitment to the service and the people using it first.

Thus, according to Evert Hughes, one of the first sociologists interested in professionalism, 'professionals profess to know better than others the nature of certain matters, and to know better than their clients what ails them or their affairs, and to offer them an esoteric service' (Hughes, 1993: 375). This is the basis of their social mandate. 'In a professional capacity a person is expected to think objectively about matters which he himself would find painful to approach in that way when they affect him personally' (p. 375). This comes together with 'the right to deviate from lay conduct in action and in thought with respect to the matter which he professes; it is an institutionalized deviation'.

'Since the professional does profess, he asks that he be trusted. Furthermore, the problems and affairs of men are such that the best of professional advice and action will not always solve them' (p. 375). While the client is asked to divulge his/her secrets, the professional is asked to do his/her best, but also to be protected from any unfortunate consequences of professional action.

This, in turn, leads to a strong gate-keeping function of professional organizations as to who can enter the profession and the training s/he needs to undertake. Finally, only the professional is authorized to say when his (and her) colleague makes a mistake (p. 376).

Hence the collective claims of a profession are dependent upon a close solidarity, upon its members constituting in some measure a group apart with an ethos of its own, which implies deep and lifelong commitments.

S/he who leaves a profession are seen as something of a renegade in the eyes of those who have remained (p. 376). Technological innovations, new conceptual knowledge and organizational changes were all geared towards enhancing knowledge and monopoly.

Detachment *and* involvement are called for at the same time, as is a balance between the universal and the particular (p. 377), both difficult to sustain and prone to creating tension. Furthermore, in some professions – such as the priesthood and I would argue in mental distress too – the professional becomes privy to 'GUILTY KNOWLEDGE', namely knowledge which is different from the usual, and entails a potentially shocking way of looking at things' (p. 289). This gives the professional the licence to *think differently* (p. 290) but also accounts in part for the slowness of professional change. Hughes suggests that a good way to learn about a specific profession is by comparative study with another profession in which similar issues arise. More specifically, he is proposing that we can understand and take care not to become too personally involved with clients who come to them with rather intimate problems' (p. 316).

I would, however, suggest that the nature of these problems requires of necessity personal involvement, as well as detachment. Hughes does not, for example, dwell at all on three central elements in British mental health work:

1 Experiencing the suffering of the other as part of everyday work. That suffering is a source of fascination, heartache, helplessness at times, and its reduction constitutes the major source of professional satisfaction.
2 Working within a welfare bureaucracy. While professionals are hired to make discretionary decisions within a context of uncertainty and lack of sufficient knowledge, welfare bureaucracies invariably attempt to treat them as any other employee, and to reduce their autonomy. Thus a contradiction is at work here. There is little doubt that working with a welfare bureaucracy is a major source of stress for professionals, yet the absence of a strong organizational backup is counterproductive not only for the professional but also for the service users and their relatives.
3 As part of the social mandate, most professional activities have mixed elements of care and control, while many professionals prefer to focus on the caring functions, which give them personal satisfaction. This has led to denial of the controlling aspects, a denial more difficult to sustain as professionals in psychiatry and social work have been lumbered with more statutory responsibilities. It has led writers such as Foucault, and service users, to argue that professionals are only fulfilling controlling functions.

The lack of *agreed* standardized solutions leads professionals in mental health to the avoidance of discussion of success or failure, which is substituted by endless discussion concerning the re-construction of the history of the client's problems. Consequently, success is replaced by whether or not the professional handled well the user and the problem (pp. 321–2).

'All professionals fail in some measure to achieve what their clients want, or think they want, of them' (p. 361). All professionals make mistakes of judgement and techniques. This is, in part, due to using knowledge that is based on a mixture of theoretical, scientific and artistic knowledge.

Thus mental distress professionals face constantly the need to live with a high level of uncertainty, ambiguity and ambivalence about their own contribution and the subject matter itself, as an integral part of their professional lives (Menzies-Lyth, 1970; Ramon, 1992).

They cope with these elements by developing the following strategies:

1 Accepting one approach and dismissing all others.
2 Accepting that their knowledge is insufficient, but is better than nothing, and therefore accepting the need to learn from others.
3 Accepting the insufficiency of knowledge, but becoming indifferent (i.e., acting as if they were technicians).
4 Blaming others and other factors (e.g., the bureaucracy, lack of resources) for what is wrong in the system.
5 Magnifying small achievements.
6 Acting as a change agent within and beyond the level of individual work; going for innovation as a way of everyday work.

THE BRITISH CONTEXT

On top of the inherent high level of ambiguity and ambivalence within all mental health professions, the current climate in which professionals are operating in Britain is full of new ambiguities, to put it mildly. It is characterized by:

● The direction of the change – from large institutions to services in the community – reflects a highly critical view of professional past tradition, especially of doctors and nurses. This has put the two groups on the defensive.
● Imposition from the political sphere, especially on those working within the public sector (the majority).

This has been particularly reflected in the increase of statutory responsibilities for psychiatrists, social workers and to a lesser extent for nurses, stricter criteria as to who is eligible for services (within either a Care Programme Approach or Care Management packages), and thus reducing eligibility for many people, while reducing the autonomy of professionals at the same time.

Yet, unlike the British government (and most other Western governments and some professionals, notably in North America), I do not look forward to a system of private mental distress services. If anything, I look in horror at the American system in terms of the benefit it offers to relatively few people and the lack of benefit to the majority of service users as a result of the fragmentation and privatization of that system. Issues concerned are:

- Imposition within the service system of adherence to managerial requirements, all of which are about curtailing the autonomy of professionals, including those which introduce clearer quality assurance mechanisms and attention to what service users and relatives are saying/wanting.
- Yet a climate of innovation and greater flexibility does exist, in which those able to work out the system can get out quite a lot for their services.
- More attention to people suffering from long-term mental distress than ever before, coupled with readiness to neglect those whose suffering can be more easily prevented is fostered by the government.
- The move away from psychiatric hospitals has benefited many of the so-called 'long, long stay' (Wainwright, 1992) but not the 'new long stay'. It is easily forgotten that this move was not planned in Britain with the 'new long stay' in mind; somehow they were supposed to cease to exist as a disturbing category. Yet many professionals and the media collude with the perception that it was/is a big failure and that most of the 'new long stay' should stay in secure units. Thus the most radical – and in my view largely positive – change of the post-war period is being re-interpreted to re-segregate and criminalize the 'new long stay', most of whom are young, more assertive, better educated, yet not less suffering than are the 'long, long stay'.

For a long time the changes have been indeed imposed by the government in Britain, and supported only by a minority in most of the helping professions, especially among psychiatrists and nurses. The objections had to do both with issues of power, autonomy, inability to perceive a system whose core will not be a hospital and perceiving its closure as critique of their own work (which it was and is), and scepticism concerning the readiness of the government to invest in community mental health facilities. Paradoxically, while craving autonomy mental distress professionals were not ready to move to community services which offer much greater autonomy – and responsibility to boot – than a hospital setting will ever offer, perhaps because the community is less 'safe' as a site of professional dominance (although rehabilitation of people with long-term mental health problems has been one of the few areas of conceptual and practice development and relative success since the 1970s (Ramon, 1990; Schulz and Greenley, 1995), rehabilitation is not a fashionable area within mental health work).

The government ignored all of what we know about how to bring change and how to motivate people in organizations for change. It did not attempt to win over the professionals to its ideas until very late in the day (in 1992, with the establishment of the mental health task force) and even then did it half-heartedly, due to its belief in a fully hierarchical management structure, a belief abandoned some time ago within the management of successful private firms, even before the guru of 'downsizing' recanted (the British government is yet to recant on this issue!).

However, if – as Jones (1996) is arguing – the aim of the government was to downgrade the autonomy of the professional classes and turn them into obedient employees, then the typical response of mental health professionals could be seen as a 'success'. For, apart from a minority, the majority within mental health professions remain only reactive – and hostile without questioning – to an aggressive government, and have not come up with alternative perspectives/frameworks, solutions to problems whose existence they do not deny.

None of the professional associations has attempted to focus its efforts on winning over professionals' minds and hearts, and most basic training programmes continue to be based in the traditional mould, in which work with continued care clients is seen as an undesirable necessity, rarely focusing on exciting new possibilities, including working with users and relatives as fully fledged partners.

Yet the success in taming the professional classes carries with it the reduction in the discretionary decision-making abilities, for which the government is employing professionals in the first place.

The introduction of the purchasers–providers split did not help to raise the morale of the majority of the professionals who found themselves described as providers. The split did nothing to re-engage them in the radical change process.

Purchasers were feted and those with financial control went into the new posts with the wish to improve the system, though often not knowing what were the needs, what needed to improve, how to go about it, and how to involve most stakeholders, including professionals, in the process. By now many of them are feeling constrained yet again, either by the pressure power of those groups which represent the past, or by the pressure to spend so much on secure facilities for so few people deemed dangerous by the moral panic which has swept Britain, making nearly everyone forget that no asylum facilities in the community were put into place when hospitals were phased out, that only few accessible drop-in services exist and even fewer of these are run by ex-users. All of these services were requested by users and by a few professionals, but were not supported by either the majority of the professionals or the government (who wanted to have it on the cheap).

Despite the centrality of professionals to the mental distress system, very little research has been focused on their activities and responses, perhaps because they are expected to somehow fall into line and because this is not an outcomes-focused research (not good value for money . . .). Research on burnout (Sullivan, 1993) reflects the stress experienced by professionals, but not its source, and tends to portray professionals as victims, a rather one-sided description.

Research on organizational change (Korman and Glennerster, 1990; Tomlinson, 1992) looks at a few key players from the perspective of their contribution to the process of organizational change, or lack of such a contribution, tending to rather simplistic analysis of power keeping strategies as the main motivation.

Existing research focused on the views and responses of professionals to the change processes of the mental health system has highlighted the passive stance taken by professionals, all of whom are intelligent and relatively resourceful people in their everyday work. The passivity seems to be formed as a defensive stance against the sense of being *unwanted as autonomous actors* by their own employer, and by other interacting organizations (Ramon, 1992). Yet the same professionals were employed principally to provide an autonomous and discretionary judgement within a highly uncertain context.

It is easy to assert that all of what was wanted of them was to control the users, deemed as deviant, and that the function of autonomous judgement is to act as a smoke-screen for this controlling function. Yes, every professional activity contains also a controlling function, in so far as collective living is in part about adherence to norms accepted by the majority and imposed on the minority. Yet many professional activities are also providing a supportive function and an attempt to understand the users.

The readiness of these professionals to accept the role designated for them by their organizations which wish to view them as any other employee within a bureaucracy can be seen as the latest coping strategy, albeit one which is self-defeating. Yet can more constructive strategies be found?

Such strategies have to enable professionals to live more comfortably with some of the ambiguities that cannot be resolved, while creating new sources for a positive use of their expertise. Establishing strategies for participatory innovation as part of everyday professional life (i.e., taking a pro-active stance, and acting as a change agent not only in at the interface with the users, but also at the organizational level) could be one such major strategy. For it to happen, new alliances between professionals, users and relatives have to be formed in which participation is allowed to grow (Romme, 1993; Ramon, 1994).

Considerable change in attitudes, training, knowledge and skills would have to take place to reach such a stage (Brandon, 1991; Segal, 1991). Most of this effort has to come from within professional groups. Yet the reinvention of mental health professionals cannot take place without the active support and pressure from users and relatives, if we aim to achieve a participatory system.

REFERENCES

Beckman, S. (1990) *Professionalization: Borderline Authority and Autonomy in Work.* In: M. Burrage and R. Torstendahl (eds), *Professionalism in Theory and History: Rethinking the Study of the Professions,* 9th edn. Beverly Hills, CA: Sage, pp. 115–138.

Brandon, D. (1991) *Implications of Normalisation Work for Professional Skills.* In: S. Ramon, *Beyond Community Care: Normalisation and Integration Work,* 9th edn. London: MIND/Macmillan.

Hughes, E. (1993) *The Sociological Eye.* New Brunswick, NJ: Transaction Books.

Illich, I. (ed.) (1968) *The Disabling Professions.* London: Marion Boyars.

Jones, C. (1996) Social work and social work educators within the context of the British New Right. Presentation to the ATSWE annual conference, 15 July.

Korman, N. and Glennerster, H. (1990) *Hospital Closure: A Political and Economic Study.* Milton Keynes: Open University Press.

Menzies-Lyth, I. (1970) *The Functioning of Social Systems as a Defence against Anxiety.* London: Tavistock.

Ramon, S. (ed.) (1990) *Psychiatry in Transition: British and Italian Experiences.* London: Pluto Press.

Ramon, S. (1992) The workers' perspective: living with ambiguity, ambivalence and challenge. In: S. Ramon (ed.), *Psychiatric Hospital Closure: Myths and Realities.* London: Chapman and Hall.

Ramon, S. (1994) Training mental health service providers in the 1990s. In: R. Leiper and V. Field (eds), *Counting for Something in Mental Health Services.* Aldershot: Avebury.

Romme, M. and Escher, S. (eds) (1993) *Accepting Voices.* London: MIND.

Schulz, R. and Greenlay, J. (eds) (1995) *Innovation in Community Care for the Severely Mentally Ill: International Perspectives.* New York: Praeger.

Segal, J. (1991) The professional perspective. In: S. Ramon (ed.), *Beyond Community Care: Normalisation and Integration Work.* London: MIND/Macmillan.

Sullivan, P. (1993) Stress and burnout in psychiatric nursing. *Nursing Standard,* 8(2): 36–38.

Tomlinson, D. (1992) *Utopia, Community Care and the Retreat from the Asylums.* Milton Keynes: Open University Press.

Wainwright, T. (1992) The changing perspective of a resettlement team. In: S. Ramon (ed.), *Psychiatric Hospital Closure: Myths and Realities.* London: Chapman and Hall.

Introduction to Chapter 9

Alec Jenner

by Chris Stevenson

In some respects, this preface is redundant in the light of the account that follows. Alec Jenner presents his own history better than I could hope to do from my brief, though memorable, encounters with him in the run-up to the Longhirst Conference and at the event itself.

Alec Jenner has had a long (as he points out) and distinguished (which he is less ready to point out) career in psychiatry. He is currently Professor Emeritus, University of Sheffield. He is a natural raconteur, and, after over forty years service to psychiatry, he has a store of stories for all palates. Alec has managed to balance his initial academic persona of biochemist with a befriending of the ideas of Ronnie Laing, who generously showed many facets of his self to Alec. He has published many papers in both 'main stream' and lesser known psychiatric journals.

Alec has been instrumental in the democratic psychiatry movement and is part of the editorial collective of the magazine *Asylum*. Perhaps, I have been most struck in my encounters with Alec and his work by the humanity that seeps out even from his standard academic writing. I have often heard psychiatric professionals speculate about who would be the best person to help them with their own (always hypothetical) distress. For those who know him, I think Alec would be top of the pops! Few people seem able to engage in a full range of human activity, from philosophy to psychiatry to partying, with such easy transitions.

All summaries are necessarily inaccurate, and the following 'sound bite' is probably more inadequate than most: Alec Jenner is a gentleman and a scholar.

9

Deconstructing over half a century of increasing involvement with psychiatry

Alec Jenner

This chapter presents, among other ideas, an approach to the thesis that much of the apparent authority of psychiatry depends on an almost hegemonic vocabulary and language. Nevertheless, the concept of 'the myth of mental illness' is itself as concretizing and dogmatic, and a slogan of a contending party. Similarly, the view that, for example, 'schizophrenia is a scientific delusion' can score illicit goals. Words have meanings within a language, to the degree that they communicate an ability to distinguish one thing, or an event, from another. Few words accurately and precisely identify things, without any ambiguity. Nevertheless, we are bound to try to produce meaningful discourse about mental states, either those like depression, undesirable for sufferers, or those like mania and psychopathy, undesirable to others. The plea is implied that we would be wise to see how distant from our ontological aims we usually have to be, and how much we should, therefore, accept necessarily political and vested interest aspects behind our own ideologies and professions.

REFLECTING PERSONALLY

When old, it is flattering to still be asked to pass on one's wisdom, and tell something of one's own life story. Whoever wanted to talk about anything more important to themselves than themselves, even if they have to deconstruct it? Yet following the invitation, there is a sinking feeling that a certain emptiness might be all that can be revealed. One, as an authority, may then be seen through!

I had always realized that an expert is someone far away from their family. The word 'expert' is interesting and might be my excuse, as it is allied, in its origins, to one who tried and learned by experience. Who would dislike the epitaph that (s)he tried to learn from experience? But what is the authority of the expert I am expected to deconstruct? Derrida's concept of Deconstruction is literary, and about words. He emphasizes the necessary contradiction between what is written and what is revealed. With that in mind, there is a case for focusing on the treachery of words. They don't, however, undermine technologies that work, for example, motor mechanics and pharmacology, but the word 'works' opens a Pandora's Box, often requiring a comment on for whom, or for what – clearly, unusual for certain purposes.

The word 'authority' is obviously etymologically related to 'author', the creator, but less clearly, but historically in fact so, to auction, augment and August, the month and imperial bearing, and hence Caesar Augustus, who clearly had a great deal of authority, as we would understand the word. Julius Caesar was given the title in 27 BC to mean 'magnificent', and the month was given his name to celebrate his greatness. As will become apparent, I suspect we all aspire to something like it, but learn to hide our egotism behind a veneer of politeness and concern for others.

Much psychopathology is the failure to continue to respectably repress ourselves. The various words related to 'authority' are all probably from the Latin *augere*, 'to create or increase'. However, ideas about the original meanings of words are more intriguing than dependable, though occasionally revealing political motives. More reliable is the realization that the meanings change and they don't just correspond with things in the world, independently of us and our social history and outlook.

To be provocative, let us consider, in the above light, the 'myth of mental illness' (Szasz, 1972). Thomas Szasz wants illness to refer to the consequences of a lesion. Humpty-Dumpty insightfully insisted a word 'means just what I choose it to mean, neither more nor less'. The word 'ill' comes from the Scandinavian group of languages. It once meant badness, even wickedness. We use it now to refer, in the mental field, to undesirable behaviours, experiences or ideas for which we do not blame the person. This led Thomas Szasz (1994) to coin another catchphrase 'Cruel Compassion', and by this, he is referring to the fact that if you say someone's views are due to a brain disease, you disenfranchise him or her. Discourse might then be as irrelevant as hoping for a speaking cure (Freud's term) for meningitis.

That view is perhaps too absolutist – it might be more difficult to persuade someone out of his mistaken views influenced by his biochemistry. However, just as some cars with defects can, with luck, be coaxed up hills, so too some psychotic persons may nevertheless be persuadable. That which, in fact, gives authority to try to persuade us is a mixture of ideology, a misleading vocabulary, money, rhetoric, dogma and evidence. The latter, evidence, is most worthy of respect. Care is certainly necessary in this field to ascertain what is the evidence, and what has been demonstrated by it. We cannot, for example, deny the evidence that drugs work, and while, certainly, that does not prove so much about the aetiology of psychoses, those results must raise the suspicion of real physical factors being involved. Everybody who has ever tried to consider the relation between body and mind knows how difficult the field is. I hold that our knowledge is never better than the technological demonstration of what works, and hopefully I will develop that idea as we go along.

I am aware that processes, in many senses of the word, work for somebody. Perhaps some central issues can be demonstrated in the best pharmacological result I ever got in many decades of exploring psychopharmacology (Hanna *et al.*, 1972). As I will explain later, as a young biochemist I became interested in abnormal mental states, which seemed to recur periodically and predictably. I came across a man whose manic depressive illness had a 48-hour rhythm over several years. The world literature contains, over the centuries, several other similar persons. Much else, which can be more objectively measured than mood, did vary with a 48-hour rhythm too, for example, the urine volume and salivary rate. Lithium carbonate stopped the cycle, and delighted the patient and his family. After three years, we gave, in a blind manner, a placebo, to be sure the continuation of lithium was justified. It was; he quickly relapsed. Was his condition best described by the epithet 'a myth of mental illness'? Was our treatment 'cruel compassion'? Compulsion was not involved, but would it have been justified?

Thomas Szasz is not opposed to the use of drugs, if that is what the client wants. He is not opposed to compulsion, as long as the psychiatrist doesn't use it in the name of medicine. To be trusted, according to Szasz, the psychiatrist should be like the Catholic priest to whom you can, without fear, confess anything, and to be convincing, the psychiatrist must demand the payment he can get from the individual. Why else care for him? Clearly, Szasz sees medical arrangements as business contracts. I agree that the mandate historically given by society to, or taken by medicine for, psychiatry, etymologically medicine of the mind, in relation to the mental health services, stretches much more questionably beyond the limits of the so-called psychoses. The wisdom of Pessoa (see Zbigniew, 1997), the leading modern Portuguese poet, is correct:

> In reality the unique critics of art and literature ought to be the psychiatrists; although they are as ignorant about these issues, and as remote from them, and what they call science, as other people, nevertheless,

when faced with mental disease they have the competence that our judgement says they have. No body of human knowledge can be built on any other bases.

No one should overlook the dangers of society psychiatrizing itself, any more than missing the point that societies defined madness first, and gave it to psychiatry, which, like other professions, tries to expand its territory. Areas of the so-called mental health field, in which there is clearly ground for considerable dispute over ownership, are obvious. There are problems associated with trying to distinguish psychopathy (better called sociopathy) from criminality. Further, is drug misuse a crime or an illness? Can psychoanalysis reduce people's explanation of behaviour to sets of deterministic psychodynamic laws, and thereby deny their freedom and responsibility, while pretending that massive amounts of training improve therapeutic skills, by making the analyst an objective observer? Their need for the law to have a register of psychotherapists, as it does of bona fide medical practitioners, seems a blatant trade unionism. These areas I will put, with so much else, on one side.

My medical background would therefore be more difficult to defend. I do agree that they present the problem of the psychologized society. Society, however, needs courts, and they need a concept of justice, largely in order to defend ownership of property, but inevitably to pronounce on responsibility, about which we know nothing. We are, therefore, doomed to play games like those of justice. In bringing up children, too, we do have to designate that which is good and bad. They, in turn, do incorporate that, and hence, if not psychopathic, do feel guilt when not complying.

Let us return to the dogmatic rejection of psychoses as illnesses, as this is the field in which I have worked most, and I want to stimulate discussion. First, I want to reassert the psychopharmacological efficacy of the major tranquillizers, as well as of lithium carbonate. This alone means that the diagnostic categories are not meaningless.

My first encounter with psychiatry was in the early 1940s. I had previously, as a young boy, felt certain that girls were rubbish, but then something happened. I was smitten by the beauty of Betty, who lived along the road. One day I called for her, but her agitated mother said she no longer wished to see me. Whilst the force of attraction may not have been as powerful in both directions, I was devastated. Then I learned that Betty had been admitted to Hanwell Asylum, now St Bernard's, Ealing, and, at one time, the hospital in which the liberal open door and no restraint advocate, John Connelly, had worked. I went to see her. She was catatonic and dishevelled, and while to me still poignantly adorable, her clothes were in wretched disarray. She took little notice of me.

If calling her state that of a mental illness was to give it a mythical title, the human problem was no myth, nor was its management easy. Further, if to call the state schizophrenic was to be a deluded partner in a *folie à deux* with psychiatrists using a meaningless term, there remains a need for a more adequate language. Here it is not possible to go very deeply into the denotation of the word meaning. Yet a statement must communicate something which allows differentiation of things. Then, to some extent, the sentences in which the word occurs have intellectual content.

The fact is that we never know everything. There is a ubiquitous ambiguity in every language, and most terms. This is illustrated, for example, by when a tree becomes a bush, or a river a stream (one cannot quite translate that into French, in which the width of the flow is irrelevant, only whether it flows into the sea or not). That does not mean the words are meaningless, nor are they useless, nor are they the right number of classes for all purposes. This aspect of language is often demonstrated by the apparently large number of words Eskimos have for snow. Nevertheless, the words we do have to hand do constrain what we are likely to think, and there is a political element involved.

Calling a mental state an illness does give some authority to doctors. Betty's problem arose before the era of chlorpromazine, when many patients didn't have their own clothes or lockers, and the beds were next to each other in massive institutions. It was also a period when gross catatonic symptoms were so much more prevalent – a fact which led me, as a young biochemist, to study catatonia, unsuccessfully, as well as to translate the leading text jointly with L. Gjessing and H. Marshall (see Gjessing, 1976). The catatonic, in fact, almost disappeared while I did so. I believe the phenothiazines were important, as well as the improved conditions of the mental hospitals, although a categorical explanation of the disappearance of the severer forms remains obscure.

Having lived through so many changes in the mental health services, I want to assert that it is very mistaken to insist that there have been no improvements. Foucault's easy dismissal of Pinel, and everyone else, seems to me little more than Gallic intellectual exhibitionism, associated with much intellectual sparkle, but little positive thinking, and no contribution of helpful suggestions about what we should do in the face of real problems. I like the French concept of '*camisol chemique*', chemical straight-jacket, to describe the phenothiazines. I am intrigued by the fact that the cerebral actions of clozepine seem to damage aspects of the classical dopamine hypothesis of schizophrenia, and even of what is the effective psychopharmacological action of the major tranquillizers. The underlying interpretation of the significance of the technology is less valid than the observation of the effectiveness. I am aware of the side effects, some of which involve permanent damage to the brain.

Having raised technology above science, I need to say how I am using the terms. In fact, here, technology is knowing what you want and how to achieve it, and science is pure knowledge, irrespective of desires. As used by me, 'science' involves the question of what does it really mean intellectually, that is, ontologically. I am asserting that we seldom know that. We know more about our own desires. Perhaps we can be helped if we try to consider some aspects of grammar, and what could, perhaps, be called their political importance. Here, I will only deal with one category of words, prepositions. Anyone trying to learn a foreign language will know how arbitrary they can be; however, I want to point out the areas where the lack of some mandatory rules does allow one to get away with less than adequate generalizations. If you, as I have, use the word 'work', and English does not demand that you follow it with a preposition, for example 'for', the *camisol chemique* may only be good, only work, 'for' the family, and not 'for' the patient. It is important 'for' clarity that 'important' should also be followed by 'for'. Not to do so assumes that we agree on what is important or good. Probably, there is a tendency to do so in physical medicine, where most would concede that broken arms and legs, cancer, and cardiac failure etc. are bad for most people. In the field of mental difficulties, agreement is less universal.

Myths, mistaken beliefs in politics, nationalism and religions make this strikingly so, telling the truth is not the supremely always defensible virtue. Father Christmas has his time and place. Further, Voltaire (see Besterman, 1971), certainly something of a sceptic, illustrates that other people's views are important for us, irrespective of their truth value. He wrote: 'I want my attorney, my tailor, my servants, even my wife, to believe in God, and I think that then I shall be robbed and cuckolded less often.' There is no doubt, either, that deviations from the hegemonic influenced sense of the time adds to the likelihood that one will be seen as being mentally ill.

That which has been written above arises in an attempt to water down the dogma of the 'myth of mental illness'. However, this must be done without concretizing matters, as does another set of catchwords: 'no twisted thought without a twisted molecule'. The latter is ridiculous, not least because most molecules are twisted, and as the adjective 'twisted' is vague in regard to ideas. The way of writing illustrates much about language too; straight is good, twisted is bad, which, to some extent, is so – certainly in the case of a ruler, but always in molecules, for example? The remark is strange, too, because it is difficult to see how the atoms we learnt about could ever bang together enough to produce, for example, the experience of jealousy. Nevertheless, there is something of that in current chemical attempts to explain the basis of, for example, paranoid ideas.

To return to the studies mentioned, the periodic conditions, this is to illustrate a simple point it took some time to grasp. As I had been taught biochemistry by a distinguished Nobel Laureate (Sir Hans Krebs), I was overwhelmed with the potential of the subject, and the validity of what I took to be the scientific method. Krebs was impressed by the possible potential of studying biological clocks, so well illustrated by the periodicity of some rare psychotic illnesses. So it was decided to do studies on the, even then, comparatively rare persons whose conditions really were clockwork-like in their recurrences. All, it was hoped, was necessary, was to show what else changed chemically with the same rhythm, and then put the pieces of the jigsaw together. The rhythms were not sociological, nor seasonal, so they must be aspects of internal chemico-physical oscillators. The scientist wants to limit the number of variables in his work, so we controlled almost everything in our patients' lives – only the clocks mattered. We forgot that violin strings oscillate at one frequency if stretched by a constant pull. There is no such thing as no environment influencing events. However, I suddenly found that moving some patients to another sociological environment stopped the cycles – perhaps the tension on the strings was different. I cannot go into this at great length, but if the patient moved with members of the nursing staff to another ward during cleaning, nothing changed. If the patient went alone to another ward and regime, there was a lengthy remission.

Here, I only want to make the point that the sociological or pharmacological effects could have been studied. What one did study was a projection of the 'scientist', not something given by the situation itself. I realized that I had picked what would make my own prejudices and wishes demonstrably true, and me an authority, hopefully using the results to argue that we could build on them, and get more money for my ideology. Extrapolation, though, began to strike me, too, as humanly inevitable. We have to learn, from limited experience, what will come next. Nevertheless, there is something political and precarious about how we are likely to do it. This sort of science depended on studying exotic examples, chosen, unconsciously perhaps, to be likely to lend support to a way of viewing matters in general.

I was imbued at work with the idea that it is all biochemistry, really. That was, unless I was angry with someone who was then clearly responsible. At home, I didn't tell my wife, nor the children, that their limbic systems were causing their behaviour. I was also impressed by how patients thought R.D. Laing's (1964) *The Divided Self* was insightful. I was, and am, confused, in this field. One should be. As Emersen (see Morley and Everelt, 1947) wrote: 'A foolish consistency is the hobgoblin of little errands, adored by little statesmen, and philosophers and divines.' However, I was the Director of a Medical Research Council Group for 'Metabolic Studies of Mental Disorders', and had a hefty mortgage to pay etc., etc. None of which is an adequate excuse for failing to see the humanistic, engaged, ideologically committed status of all human beings. This led to a set of ideas which may be relevant to the field of the Authority of Psychiatry.

First, the pragmatism I have mentioned above, and the obvious fact that human beings are all trying to find a place of some importance for themselves. As social animals, the respect of others is desired, indeed, to perceive one has it, is almost a necessary vitamin for a healthy mental life. The problem is that the importance for the self and the respect of others has something of the paranoid paradox about it. Most of us learn to discipline ourselves to take diplomatic steps to get our own way and respect. You do what is necessary to become a professor of psychiatry and fool yourself that it brings great respect. Much of the game is played in terms of trade unions, even nationalism, gender allegiances, religious, and arbitrary professional groupings. Much is produced in relation to the game and the prescribed rules, not least the unwritten one, known by the wise, which says that the art of politics is winning, not protesting. The codicil adds that the equipment and size of the opposing army is an important factor in terms of strategy, and, further, that there is a sense in which human beings are more strikingly ethicizing than ethical.

Most, to the same extent, almost instinctively know all this, but we are still vulnerable to *Schadenfreude*, anger, hurt, jealousies, anxiety and depression, and we cannot just play cards, especially when it seems we, ourselves, are the ones that never or seldom win. In the middle of all this income is a striking measure of success, respect and power. I have enjoyed, as a medic, more than I would be able to defend, when compared to a social worker or nurse, even if I am a pauper compared to the leaders of Britain's denationalized industries, of which my share was sold too cheaply! The reality of a capacity for compassion cannot be denied, and certainly, the development of all manner of mutually supporting groups is ubiquitous, like the identity given by supporting football teams. The fact is that in much of the game, arguments are powerful, but seldom overwhelmingly logical, as distinct from being an aspect of political hegemony. Nevertheless, you can fool some of the people a lot of the time, despite the mad nature of so much argument. Indeed, many are being polite because it pays, while the radicals see gain in criticism. The upheaval to make it better is often so unlikely to be practical, just as the revolutions in the world can result in laments like that of Mme Jeanne Manon Roland, who cried before her death at the guillotine, 'O Freedom, what crimes are committed in thy name' (quoted by Macaulay in his essay on Mirabeau).

Having, in fact, written the above for a book organized by nurses, I do have to say that the defence of my privileges is difficult. When I first went to a mental hospital, the nurses wore strange outfits and stood to attention when the medical superintendent did his round. They were much less well educated than the doctors, even the poor medical specimen who didn't actually run mental asylums (the nurses did that, for much less cash). Now all professions are better educated, and much more able to argue about matters with the medical staff. Indeed, much of their training is much more relevant to what they are doing, though each plays the multi-diplomatic game to some effect. The truth is that the really useful knowledge in all fields is limited. Psychiatry's trump card is only about four or five types of drugs, and its dominance is older than they are. Perhaps there is little need for such different professions. The advantage, of course, of the colonizer of a field, is obvious, but while not occupying the position of power, the colonized are given the privilege of implying they wouldn't have acted like that! The pleasure of paranoia is given to them quite cheaply. On the other hand, it is abundantly clear that psychiatry does have a category for those who feel they are being persecuted when they are not, but no place for those who are being ill-treated without noticing. They are among the most likeable people! I think that many, called schizophrenic, passionately notice, and are depressed by the madness of the world, but they fail to see that they have to live in it. Opting out and protesting etc., etc. only makes it all worse for themselves. I believe the major tranquillizers help them to reflect peacefully enough to compromise with the reality that they, perhaps rightly enough, dislike. A reality which is sometimes similarly rejected when they stop taking their medication although these 'relapses' could also be withdrawal phenomena.

I do not think that the reflection is completely conscious, any more than I think we are aware of the control from outside affecting our thoughts and behaviour. They complain, perhaps more insightfully than we do, of the real sites of the locus of control. These all represent fundamental states of being human. Everyone needs help to find a respected place at the table with the rest of us, or to live in another unreal world. I understand that it might be so among the Mapucci Indians of Chile, that in some tribes apparently schizophrenic women are made priestesses, and do not have further episodes. Were they, too, in need of power and authority, not alienation and isolation? Clearly, I feel those who can do most to make the other feel at home should have most authority, even if, in some cases, the conflict level is hardly resolvable, other than with drugs. The achievements of pharmacology, of the neurochemical studies of brain function, and now increasingly of molecular biology and sociobiology, are quite undeniable. Nevertheless, politics, sociology and psychology cannot yet be subsumed in those other sciences. Further, there may be changes in how we can perceive physicalism, and that may displease many Authorities.

REFERENCES

Besterman, T. (ed.) (1971) *Voltaire – Philosophical Dictionary.* Harmondsworth: Penguin.

Gjessing, R. (1976) *Somatology of Periodic Catatonia* (translated and edited by L. Gjessing, H. Marshall and F.A. Jenner). Oxford: Pergamon Press.

Hanna, S.M., Jenner, F.A., Pearson, I.B. *et al.* (1972) The therapeutic effect of lithium carbonate in a patient with a 48-hr periodic psychosis. *British Journal of Psychiatry*, **121**: 271–280.

Laing, R.D. (1964) *The Divided Self.* Harmondsworth: Penguin.

Moriey, C. and Everelt, L.D. (eds) (1947) *Bartlett's Familiar Quotations.* Boston: Little, Brown and Company.

Szasz, T. (1972) *The Myth of Mental Illness.* St Albans: Granada.

Szasz, T. (1994) *Cruel Compassion.* New York: John Wiley & Sons.

Zbigniew, K. (1997) *Fernando Pessoa: Voices of a Lamadie Soul.* London: Routledge.

Part Two

Complementary and critical voices

Introduction

Phil Barker and Chris Stevenson

The issues raised in Part One were traditional: freedom, liberty, control, race, identity and the nature of human helpfulness. In addition to how we might relate – intellectually – to such phenomena, the chapters also included allusions to how people process such experiences: what they *do* with such experiences at a human level. In Part Two, we continue the exploration of the 'what' and 'how' of psychiatric power and authority, both questions that might lend themselves to a consideration of 'why'. Whether or not the authors in Part One addressed 'why-ness' to the satisfaction of the readers, only the readers, themselves, can judge. Our original intention was to provoke. We heard a distant echo, which sounded like Socrates ringing down the centuries, challenging us to explain ourselves. What, exactly, was our concern about power and authority? What are the origins of our anxiety concerning these two specific dimensions of interpersonal and social exchange? Being modest, uncertain – or, hopefully, both – we chose some of the foremost voices in the world of psychiatry, social work and psychology – to whom we felt an affiliation, if not an attachment – to represent us. We added, for very good measure, a voice from the dispossessed: a representative of all bestowed with the dubious honour of 'patienthood'. These voices spoke for us. In retrospect, we believe that they reflected well our inconsistencies, our uncertainties, our fervently held beliefs and also some of our *feelings*.

In Part Two, we cast our net more widely, over potentially deeper waters. Here, we admit not only more of those who appear, in our estimation, to represent some of our anxieties, but also some who appear – at least on first reading – to oppose us. Just as the mirror exhibits everything that we are *not* – our re-flection – so too might some of these authors, by their differing slants on power and authority, reflect our own positions, whatever they might be. Again, the reader will be the judge of whether or not this reflection is realized.

In Part Two, we have brought together a group of voices, which is similarly disparate, and equally discordant. Again, perhaps, what they have in common is their struggles with uncertainty; their tussles with the complex order that is the human experience, and psychiatry's attempts to contain it, locate it within some conceptual boundary and, hopefully, to understand it.

Little, if anything has been said so far about the complex set of orders that represent families, far less the wider community to which people belong. We may have been guilty, for far too long, of acting *as if* the individual patient (*sic*) was a wholly interpersonally isolated phenomenon. Everyday discourse – not to mention soap operas – demolishes that mythology. Individuals are embedded in complex social realities, which they help define, but which also define them. What understanding does psychiatric power and authority have of such specialized social contexts?

Although modern psychiatry made its name – at least in the lay public arena – through contemplation and the couch, little of that isolating world of introspective analysis remains. It was overtaken, at least momentarily, by an appreciation that even personal dialogue occurs in an interpersonal milieu. Several authoritative voices have argued that it occurs best, in the chaotic, everyday discourse called – perhaps inappropriately – *everyday* discourse. Given the longstanding interest in the potentialities of the therapeutic community, we have included a chapter that addresses some of its core themes and principles.

For at least the past twenty years, we have been engrossed in an ideological struggle with the concept of 'community care'. This ill-titled piece of altruistic theory has stimulated all manner of adherents, prophets and soothsayers. It has also provided a solid basis for its own deconstruction: that the 'community' does *not* care, being its original and perhaps final downfall. Such doubts – and pragmatic admissions of 'reality' – have stimulated an appreciation of the values of *asylum*: values which we appear to have, so readily, overlooked, in our lemming rush to community care. A chapter that reflected on asylum – as a human virtue – has, therefore, been included.

The layperson might assume that beneath all these philosophical and ideological tussles, lies some core ambition – perhaps instinct – to benefit, or even simply care for, our fellow beings. This implies a culture of compassion. Such an implication may well be wide of the everyday mark of psychiatric reality. However, it did seem appropriate to profile the compassionate voice, and we are well served here by someone who not only connects us to the layperson's notion of *care*, but who also serves as a conduit across philosophical cultures, if not time itself.

Threaded through many of the dialogues in the text, is the vexatious issue of classification, labelling and diagnosis. Their ideological kin are, of course, the philosophical assumptions that helped them through the birthing process. We addressed some of the key arguments for individual liberty and against, allegedly flawed, if not also stigmatizing, diagnosis. As a conclusion to Part Two we offer the other side of that well-worn coin: theoretical and philosophical arguments in favour of classification, as *part* of our search for understanding and control over madness. There are longstanding arguments in favour of the *responsible* use of power and authority in psychiatry: here we remind ourselves of the nature, and supporting rationales, for such arguments.

Introduction to Chapter 10

Jane Andrews, Jim Birch, Alex Reed, Glynnis Spriddell and Chris Stevenson
(the North Shields Family Team)

by Chris Stevenson

The group who have written this paper have an alias. In another world, they are known as the North Shields Family Team. The team came together in 1993 as a result of a confluence of circumstances. The original team members, Jim Birch, Alex Reed and I, had known each other and of each other's interest in family work for some time. We were working in community psychiatry (J.B.) and as community mental health team co-ordinators, with a background in psychiatric nursing (A.R. and C.S.). As we bumped into each other in the arenas of psychiatric systems, it became clear that, between the three of us, there was a shared dissatisfaction with the kind of family approaches in which we had become practised. There was a collective sense that the structural and strategic manipulation of families by the active therapist was passé. Instead there was the tantalizing possibility of introducing a new, respectful approach to meeting with families, drawing on the work of Tom Andersen, Harlene Anderson and Harry Goolishian, Lynn Hoffman and other 'therapists' who were siting themselves within the post-modern turn. Jim and Alex were able to engineer the space to devote one morning a week to family sessions, although this had a profound effect on the amount of clinical work they had to do in the rest of the week. I was lucky enough to be part of an academic institution that valued the connection between university and industry, which valued academics who were practitioners also. Family meetings at 26A Hawkey's Lane, North Shields began. We were joined briefly by Sue Owens, and then by Nancy Bineham, before a social work colleague, Glynnis Spriddell, recruited herself to the team. More recently Steve Nash has joined the team as a valuable and valued member.

Contemporaneously to the forming of the team, we were lucky enough to acquire some funding for a research studentship from the University of Sunderland where I was teaching at that time. Jane Andrews was recruited to the team with a brief of exploring the families' perceptions of the process of the particular (and peculiar) meetings we established in order that we had an evaluation of our work; an evaluation which was conducted in a manner which was mindful of the power implicit in the creation of the research and researcher, in the same way that our practice was mindful of the privileged position of the professional team.

As the team has established itself clinically, we have been invited to present our work for different organizations, including Mental Health North, the British Psychological Society Psychotherapy Branch, Royal College of Psychiatrists Philosophy Section, and to engage in training workshops, locally and nationally, for different disciplines. The team members have individually and collectively produced many papers for professional journals in the five-year period of their working together.

10

Context and power in family meetings

Jane Andrews, Jim Birch, Alex Reed,
Glynnis Spriddell and Chris Stevenson

Family 'experts' and family members can be heard as engaging one another in ways which authorize the professionals' story whilst, at the same time, dis-attending to the way this authority is being constructed. Reflective practices can enquire into this construction of authority.

In thinking about this chapter we[1]are faced with a paradox. We want to write about the construction of power in meetings between psychiatry staff and psychiatry service users. We find ourselves, however, writing in an academic publication and using an exclusive professional language. If our text is that psychiatric workers should strive to examine the balance of power between service users and staff then we may already have failed in this ambition through the privileged position of writing for a publication that our clients will not read, and through the inaccessibility to our clients of the professional grammar we are accustomed to using. If we are to dispense with staff authority, through which powers do we do this? It seems that we are claiming to do this from the very authority which comes from speaking as professionals. We use our authorized voice to deny our authority. Difficulties of this order have been described by Derrida (1967/1978) as deconstruction. The term has a precise meaning, indicating that some posited underlying structure in human affairs is found to break down if applied to itself.

Derrida first described the problem in anthropology, where the ambition to generate culture-neutral descriptions of alien cultures broke down because those descriptions had to be situated in the language of the observing culture and so necessarily lost their neutrality. The general story of deconstruction is the attempt to erase an oppressive element of discourse, only to discover that element reappearing in different dress to frustrate the 'solution'. We will not be dismayed by this difficulty, but will regard it as constitutive of language as a social event which can never encompass all-there-is. Birch (1995) has drawn attention to a positive account of deconstruction in talk about therapy, arguing that it highlights those areas where professional discourse is struggling at the edge of understanding. Our response for now will be to accept that deconstruction means we can have nothing final to say about authority in family meetings, but neither will it invite us to silence.

As team members we share a value system. The story we tell each other about this is that we believe our work should be emancipatory. We do not call on any external authority for this belief, instead emancipation is for each of us part of our 'final vocabulary' (Rorty, 1980), a valued aim without which we could no longer describe ourselves as who we are. We pursue this project in many ways, in our hope that people can escape the subjugation which comes from stigmatizing talk of 'mental illness'; in our hope that persons caught up in hostile conversations can find more respectful interactions; and in our hope that a person can transcend oppressive narratives which invite marginalization or disenfranchisement.

These views also advise us to be cautious. Psychiatry staff are powerful too. Most of us assume statutory powers to deprive an individual of his or her liberty under the Mental Health Act, but we all come to meetings with the informal authority of 'experts', and with the opportunity to engage oppressively with family members.

When meeting with families we try to remain aware of our working context and its capacity to dignify our accounts of the world and to demean the accounts of family members. Psychiatry and related disciplines have established a hegemony amongst commentaries on the lives of persons. We try to keep in mind this assumed authority and to question it repeatedly. This ambition is not easy to realize. Although we are a diverse group we have all, to different extents, been accultured into the assumption of professional authority and have to work hard to step outside of this. Professional authority does not always welcome challenge. Staff in psychiatry services tend to value those elements of their life stories which emphasize working hard and making personal sacrifices to achieve qualifications. They enter into a professional grammar and this manifests their entry into a professional life where colleagues speak a language that tends to exclude the uninitiated. This is a seductive Freemasonry which does not invite critical enquiry.

Why should we bother about our authority? Lord Acton's caution that power tends to corrupt and that absolute power tends to corrupt absolutely seems to us to apply beyond what is ordinarily thought of as politics. Some experimental psychologists have thought past their own conventional positions of authority to enquire into interactions under authority. Milgram (1974) showed that a majority of ordinary people are willing to subject a stranger to pain or danger if acting under authority. Haney *et al.* (1973) showed that allocating roles of guard and prisoner to unexceptional psychology students led to escalating oppression on the part of 'guards' to the extent that his experiment had to be terminated prematurely. The issue of authority in relation to psychotherapies as a whole is dealt with in detail by Masson (1989).

We are concerned to remain aware of our position of power in relation to those with whom we meet. At its most basic, this amounts to a concern that we should not be defining or specifying the lives of those we talk with. Also we see a failure to examine accounts of our authority in our work as a form of censorship – closing off staff talk or family talk which might lead to more fruitful revisions of difficult stories.

REVISING THE AUTHORITY OF THE THERAPY LANGUAGE GAME

With regard to family meetings, we are attracted to Wittgenstein's (1953) proposal of the 'language game' as a means of understanding what happens between persons brought together in talk. That is to say, we first assume that we meet around a set of implicit rules which specify who can say what to whom, and what their talk can be taken to mean. For instance if, in the therapy language game, a staff member says to a family member, 'How are you?' a polite, 'Fine thank you, and how are you?' is not usually acceptable. Equally a staff member who replies, 'Not so well, I'm afraid. My marriage is going through a bad time just now' is also stepping outside the grammar. The conventions of the therapy language game require that service users talk about their personal problems whilst staff maintain a silence on their own problems.

From a different perspective, an observer who did not initially know the identities of the parties in a meeting would quickly work this out. A person who says, 'Please tell me what I can do about this problem,' is a service user, and a person who says, 'I think the inter-generational boundaries in this family are too loose,' is on the staff. This discriminatory grammar will also be evident around the use of the technology. 'I wonder if we should swap chairs now?' or 'Is there some way in which you would like to use the video-recording?' are the enquiries of staff members.

Of course the language game described thus could be seen as entirely deterministic. There could be a finite number of grammars which remain fixed through time. This does not fit well with most persons' experience of life with others, where change and surprise can feature at any time. We find relief in this notion of change and surprise, in that we no longer have to strive for the perfect therapy. We are attracted to the idea of a therapy language game which evolves with our own professional development, with changes in thinking which we hear about from our peers, and with the loss of our equilibrium which we gratefully receive from the service users we meet.

If we have a story about this changing therapy language game it will owe much to Pearce and Cronen's (1980) dramaturgical model. We value the idea that when we meet with service users we, and they, start with individual 'scripts' of how such a meeting might proceed. We also value the idea that these scripts get dynamically rewritten as all the parties in the meeting try to find ways of making their projects fit together comfortably. A consequence of this idea is that we must change if those who come to speak with us are changing.

REVISING THE AUTHORITY OF TECHNOLOGY

The video screen and the one-way screen are technologies which have become embedded in family therapy practice. Like any technology, they can be experienced as a source of liberation, or of subjugation. Our team has access to both these technologies and we find ourselves increasingly enquiring into how we debate their use with family members. Our contact with the work of Andersen (1990) has accentuated this tendency.

Family members, at their first meeting, will be introduced to persons and practices for which they will have had no prior guidance on conventional responses and no opportunity to have rehearsed a range of responses of their own. They will probably have had experience of a consultation process of some sort – few people, for example, will be unfamiliar with the conduct of a general practitioner. They are much less likely to have had a consultation video-recorded or to have encountered the one-way screen. They meet with a group of staff who can appear blasé about these technologies. We try to remember this, and to see the interviewing suite as newcomers might see it. We are helped by not having an invariant regime for our meetings. This means that we are able to enquire into the comfort of family members; to give them options on how the screen is used; to invite them to consider how and when they might meet the whole team; to allow them to consider the video-recorder and its possible uses.[2]

Paradoxically this deliberate weakening of our authority around the technology leaves us feeling liberated by diverse family values rather than constrained by our loss of dictat. We find that the form of our meetings has become diverse, just as the families we meet are diverse. We have a sense now that these first negotiations about the structure of meeting is our work with a family, every bit as much as later talk about problems and solutions. Indeed these first discussions seem to be a way of establishing the authority of family members which enables later talk of problems and solutions to be owned in partnership between staff and family.

REVISING THE AUTHORITY OF PROFESSIONAL SECRECY

Staff language, the architecture of the 'viewing' suite, and the recording technology invite a culture of staff secrecy. Team member's backgrounds may be various, but we each bring with us a version of a professional cult of secrecy. This culture invites us to speak secretly of family members in a language which they would scarcely follow even if they were to overhear – a circumstance which staff learn to regard as bad practice. One staff myth about this secret talk is that it enables them to say what they 'really' feel about their clients. We invite the reader to see this construction of staff talk as being similar to that of gossip, so it is not surprising that what staff 'really' feel can sound critical, censorious, scathing, or objectifying. We prefer to think that this talk is simply the talk which is inevitably constructed within the language game of gossip. (A person joining a gossip circle who says ennobling things about the absentee under discussion plainly does not understand the rules.) Screen technology can add to the exclusiveness of staff talk. Video-tapes will typically be discussed when families are no longer in the vicinity of the work place. Most of our team first encountered the one-way screen as the barrier behind which the therapist retreated for learned discussions to which family members were not privy. Even what the family might be permitted to hear of the discussions afterwards might be carefully contrived.

We find we cannot describe this use of secrecy as emancipatory. Andersen's (1990) experiment with alternatives to traditional staff talk has inspired us into change. Andersen describes the frustration and discomfort of a team of therapists with their experience of professional gossip behind the one-way screen. Their solution was to switch the lights and sound in their interviewing suite and to invite the family to listen to the team's discussion. Our team practice is based on this sharing of staff talk and, like the Andersen team, we find that our talk carries greater esteem for our families (and perhaps for ourselves) when we are being overheard. We still speak together as a team after meeting a family, but we find that the quality of this discussion has changed. We tend now to comment on our experience from the position of therapist or team member; on how we found this comment helpful, or this other comment puzzling; on the discovery of some personal experience which impinges on our freedom to think effectively; or on talk which seemed to have closed down a conversation.

The members of our team, happily subject to normal human frailty, continue to engage in staff gossip from time to time. We find that we do less of it, that it has lost some of its satisfaction. We can now label this form of discourse and so weaken the sense that this is 'really' how we feel about family members. Often we can then notice professional prejudices which have guided our thinking or our talk about a family, and naming the prejudice can often lead to a shift which enables us to discover some new and fruitful direction.

REVISING THE AUTHORITY OF RESEARCH

A dominant narrative in health services demands that practice should be 'evidence-based'.[3] The implication of this position is that we should subject our practice to some form of research in order to justify what we do. The researcher is encultured into the languages and practices that will lead to her or his work becoming acceptable within the community of researchers. These languages and practices are concerned with reducing complex personal accounts to simpler stories which follow the grammar of cause and effect. The process of knowledge generation thus subjugates the views of the researched to the needs of the research community.

Research as a subjugation narrative fits poorly with our wish to give an account of our work as emancipatory. We take the position that our need to describe our practice reliably should not be achieved at the expense of the right of family members to develop their own way of speaking of their lives. To this end our research aims to tell the story of the co-evolving accounts of staff and family members as they talk together over time. This approach also requires us to think of our researcher (J.A.) as inevitably a part of the network of interactions through which staff and family meanings are co-constructed, and therefore part of her own research. Unlike the traditional researcher, she cannot sustain the fiction of standing outside her study, as an 'objective' authority.

REFLECTIVE PRACTICE AS A REVISION OF AUTHORITY

Andersen (1990) has described his work as moving towards a reflective practice. As we revise our own practice in this direction we recognize in our own work many of the elements of change described by him. We are less interested now in theoretical talk, preferring direct descriptions of what we have seen or heard. What we do say is offered speculatively often offering a choice of accounts any or all of which we indicate can be left unused. We do not assume that we immediately know how to begin our work together, and we regularly invite comment from our families on how comfortable they are with how we are proceeding.

We find that our focus has shifted from family to therapist-plus-family, and then to team-plus-therapist-plus family: in this shift we find ourselves speculating on what we bring to the meeting in terms of personal and professional stories.

AUTHORITY: REPRISE AND DECONSTRUCTION

Our account began with a project to examine and redraft accounts of power in therapy. For a therapist who takes a positivist position there is much that is uncertain or provisional in the way we describe our work with families. We are no longer saying such things as, 'This is our theory of family problems,' or, 'These are the stages in our therapy.' We do not offer formulae for understanding or action. From our point of view we seem to be more assured in our uncertainty, more secure in our fallibility, to the extent that we might now characterize our uncertainty and fallibility as – authoritative. Our imagined erasure of authority from our practice has generated this chapter, where we could be said to be speaking with authority. Our project to establish family meetings which are neutral for authority is thus deconstructed. Relieved, we will begin again.

EMPOWERMENT THAT IS NOT PROBLEMATIC IS NOT EMPOWERMENT

We thought to end this chapter with the comments of a person who has used our service. Mention has been made above of the interviews J.A. has been undertaking in her research. Participant K was willing to have some of his observations published, and we thank him for this.

We are aware of the issue of editorial control here. We cannot publish an entire transcript of a discussion about the family team in a brief paper. Even if we could, how do we choose which one of many such transcripts should be published? Our approach to this difficulty has been to become interested in our editorial activity. At first we sought to report those comments by K which endorsed our view that we have been engaged in a revision of authority in our work. For example:

> K: When this situation [reflective conversations with the team] first developed, I felt as though I had no rights in this situation at all – because of my background, and what had gone on before – I felt I had no input into the situation. Now, as the situation progressed, I realized that if anything was going to be done – it had to be me, and it developed in me an attitude towards the situation – I mean I have actually evolved a possible solution to it as well – which I don't know if it will happen. ....

JA: Do you have any idea what enabled you to feel that – that your voice could be heard, so to speak?

K: It's just that when I've been ill before – nobody's listened to my point of view. I wasn't ill this time – compared to what I have been – I've never had my point of view respected and, as I say, it gave me confidence to believe in it.

JA: Right, so that was an important feature for you?

K: Yes . . . yes.

JA: Thinking back to when you first came – did you have any thoughts about what to expect?

K: Well yes I did. I assumed the exercise was all about steam-rollering me again – and it wasn't – which is what it usually was in the past. I was pleasantly surprised in that respect.

Finishing on such a note might carry the implication that we think we have 'cracked' the problem of authority in therapeutic work – that we have exemplified a process of final emancipation. We find such a conclusion fits poorly with our view that the issue of authority is always problematical. We prefer to finish our chapter with a comment from K which draws attention to the way in which the ghost of authority can always revisit any account of empowerment in a relationship scripted as therapeutic.

K: As I say, I approached the whole thing with some prejudice and I'm grateful for the fact that there wasn't any advice given – that's the beauty of it. In fact to give advice would be wrong . . . the people must be allowed to make up their own minds. No, I don't think advice should be given – the world is full of people wanting to advise you about your life, but that's not the right way to do it. They adopted the right approach with that . . . the way is to bring out the solution with people – which they did do with us.

JA: I was wondering if you had any ideas about how you think they did that?

K: Well, I suppose they are trained to steer your thoughts in that direction, although you're not conscious of it happening . . .

NOTES

1 'We' will refer to the members of the family team in this chapter.

2 See Birch (1990) for an account of the unexamined issues involved in drafting the 'consent' form.

3 Whilst this demand seems self-evidently virtuous it is hard not to notice that the application of family work in adult general psychiatry, the value of which is established beyond argument, remains marginalized and impoverished. Clearly if one wishes to promote some area of practice it is not sufficient to bring forth evidence, one must also engage in some other, political, dialogue.

REFERENCES

Andersen, T. (1990) *The Reflecting Team: Dialogues and Dialogues about the Dialogues.* Broadstairs, Kent: Borgmann Publishing.

Birch, J. (1990) The context-setting function of the video consent form. *Journal of Family Therapy,* **12**: 281–286.

Birch, J. (1995) Chasing the rainbow's end and why it matters: a coda to Pocock, Frosh, and Larner. *Journal of Family Therapy,* **17**: 219–228.

Derrida, J. (trans. A. Bass) (1978) *Writing and Difference.* Chicago: University of Chicago Press (from Derrida, J. (1967) *L'Ecriture et la différence.* Paris: Editions du Seuil).

Haney, C. *et al.* (1973) Interpersonal dynamics in a simulated prison. *International Journal of Criminology,* **1**: 69–97.

Masson, J. (1989) *Against Therapy.* London: Collins.

Milgram, S. (1974) *Obedience to Authority: an Experimental View.* London: Tavistock.

Pearce, W.B. and Cronen, V. (1980) *Communication, Action and Meaning: the Creation of Social Realities.* New York: Praeger.

Rorty, R. (1980) *Philosophy and the Mirror of Nature.* Oxford: Basil Blackwell.

Wittgenstein, L. (trans. G. Anscombe) (1953) *Philosophical Investigations.* Oxford: Basil Blackwell.

Introduction to Chapter 11

Alex Reed

by Chris Stevenson

Alex Reed's first professional qualification was as a psychiatric nurse. However, his search for the alternative in psychiatry soon took him to the Henderson Hospital. The Henderson is run along the principles of a therapeutic community and this may well have awakened his first concerns with psychiatric authority. Alex followed a circuitous route into community psychiatric nursing, eventually taking on the role of a community mental health team leader and working at present as a nurse practice supervisor within Newcastle City Health Trust. Alex is a co-founder, and valued member, of the North Shields Family Team.

Alex has steadfastly maintained an interest in families. He trained as a systemic practitioner at the Kensington Consultation Centre, London, and the University of Northumbria, where he now teaches into the Diploma/MA in systemic practice. He is undertaking work towards a doctorate, researching the ways in which the boundary between hospital and community can be eroded by offering in-patients 'reception meetings'. These meetings involve the patient and invited members of the social network (professionals and others), and are a forum where stories about events leading up to admission can be discussed, where the cares and concerns around coming into and being in hospital can be addressed.

Alex has an ongoing preoccupation with the nature of power within psychiatric systems. This is apparent in his preference to research and publish in the area of power relations. He and I co-edited a special edition of the *Journal of Psychiatric and Mental Health Nursing* in 1996 which reviewed post-modernity within psychiatric nursing, with special reference to power. Alex has exposed some of the problematic areas of practice, e.g., lying clients, through his preference to refract existing psychiatric frameworks of understanding through the prism of multiple realities. Recently, Alex was awarded a Florence Nightingale Study Grant, which allowed him to spend five weeks in Finland in dialogue with psychiatric practitioners about power in a different psychiatric culture.

11

Manufacturing a human drama from a psychiatric crisis: crisis intervention, family therapy and the work of R.D. Scott

Alex Reed

INTRODUCTION

As the shift towards community care has gathered momentum in Britain during the 1980s and 1990s there has been an increase in public anxieties about how psychiatric services are responding to people identified as mentally ill. The failure of central government to provide adequate funding for services has exacerbated public concerns that people with severe difficulties have been left to fend for themselves, sometimes with disastrous consequences. Media coverage over this period has tended to both reflect and provoke these anxieties by characterizing people with mental health problems as dangerous, unpredictable and irresponsible (Johnstone, 1994). In response, legislative initiatives have been introduced which strengthen the surveillance and coercive aspects of psychiatry's social function. While these initiatives were introduced with the aim of allaying public concern, they may also have the effect of generating further anxiety by unintentionally confirming the stereotypical perceptions of the 'mentally ill' as dangerous and irresponsible.

Our practice as mental health nurses is inevitably influenced by these powerful sociocultural discourses about mental illness. The relationships we form with individual service-users, their families and our professional colleagues are strongly influenced by these dominant beliefs and attitudes, and the political and legislative framework which has been erected on the basis of them. A number of commentators (Birch, 1991;

Johnstone, 1994; Parker *et al.*, 1995) have explored the relationship between these wider cultural perspectives about mental illness and professional practice, and in his writings R.D. Scott (1973a) has analysed the constraining effects on psychiatric practice of these dominant cultural beliefs and attitudes. Scott also discusses the disabling processes that can occur when problems of living become defined as medical or psychiatric in nature, the 'closure' that occurs between the person who is labelled as ill and their wider social context, and the barrier to effective therapeutic intervention which is constructed as a consequence of this. These ideas will be discussed in some detail in this article, as they provided the theoretical rationale for the 24-hour crisis service which Scott and his co-workers developed.

BACKGROUND

Dr Scott is a psychiatrist who initially trained in individual psychotherapy and began to study family therapy in 1960, participating in regular seminars on communications theory and family studies in schizophrenia at the Tavistock Clinic in London, together with colleagues such as Laing, Esterson, Cooper and Lee, who were at the forefront of applying these ideas in the UK (Clay, 1996). Scott also led a research team which carried out intensive studies based on their clinical work with families using a systemic perspective (Scott and Ashworth, 1967, 1969).

These early articles by Scott and his co-workers were of their time in the sense that they were characterized by a concern with aetiological factors associated with family dynamics. However, just as he had made an earlier shift from using individual therapy to a family orientated approach, Scott later continued to widen the theoretical lens through which he viewed psychiatric disorder to include sociocultural concerns. By the early 1970s Scott had, to use his own words, 'emerged out of the family hinterland into the light of day, and seen how many abnormalities in family relationships are based on the cultural image of mental illness' (Scott, 1973b: 65). Over this period he continued to apply these new ideas in his general psychiatric practice (Scott, 1973a, 1980; Scott and Starr, 1981), and the understanding that he developed about the significance of cultural beliefs about mental illness encouraged his shift towards the development of a community orientated crisis-intervention service.

CULTURAL BELIEFS ABOUT MENTAL ILLNESS AS A 'TREATMENT BARRIER'

In order to understand how particular beliefs and attitudes towards mental illness have come to be predominant within contemporary Western society, it is helpful to consider the history and development of these ideas. Rosen (1994) offers an account of the ways in which perceptions of those viewed as insane have altered over time. He suggests that in prehistoric times society was organized into small communities with systems of extended kinship and that people who displayed strange or unusual behaviour would tend to remain included rather than be expelled. Such people were often regarded as having special spiritual abilities or gifts. Rosen argues that as a consequence of the widespread influence of Greek civilization during the fourth and fifth centuries, the Western Intellectual Tradition became established which was characterized by the elevation of the concept of Reason. It was during this era that madness came to be regarded as a human failing rather than a state of heightened spirituality, and those people who were seen to be insane tended to be expelled from communities or allowed to wander, with no particular provision made for them. During the period of the Enlightenment in the late seventeenth and eighteenth centuries, the ideals of Rationality and Reason became further elevated, and it was during this period that the practice of locking away the mad in purpose-built institutions began. This is the period described by the French philosopher Michel Foucault as 'the Great Confinement' (Rosen, 1994: 130).

Foucault argued that the inhabitants of these institutions did not come to be regarded as 'sick' until the end of the eighteenth century, when ideas about the moral treatment of people seen principally as weak or maladjusted gave way to medical understandings of insanity, and the birth of psychiatry as a specialist branch of medicine (Parker *et al.*, 1995). The eventual dominance of the medical-psychiatric perspective was finally achieved with the advent of major tranquillizers in the 1950s. The effectiveness of these drugs has generally been regarded as a fundamental advance in the treatment of the mentally ill which created the possibility of community care in its present form (Parker *et al.*, 1995). The notion of madness as brain disease has subsequently reigned supreme. It is debatable, for instance, whether the radical critique of orthodox psychiatry provided by R.D. Laing and others (Laing, 1967) in the 1960s and early 1970s impacted greatly on mainstream psychiatric practice. In relation to the field of psychiatric nursing, some recent evidence regarding the dominance of the biological perspective is provided by a study undertaken by the Sainsbury Centre for Mental Health (Warner *et al.*, 1997). In this study a number of psychiatric nurses working in different Trusts in England were asked to identify the specific skills that they felt mental health nurses needed in their work with people with severe mental health problems. All of the nurses who participated in the research identified dealing with medication as a key area of nursing practice, but few mentioned specific psychotherapeutic interventions such as cognitive therapy, and none mentioned family therapy.

In Western society the dominant societal beliefs about persons who are characterized as mentally ill therefore include the idea that psychiatric disorder occurs as a consequence of biochemical or genetic factors; that the problems are located 'inside' of the individual; and that the person who is afflicted lacks 'insight' into his or her true situation and lacks responsibility or personal agency (Scott, 1973a, 1973b). Once a diagnosis of mental illness is awarded to the individual, the problems are generally seen as unrelated to the social context in which the person has been living their life.

When an individual is defined as mentally ill in this way, 'illness' comes to be seen as an aspect of their identity, so that we describe a person as a 'schizophrenic' or an 'agoraphobic' in such a way that no space exists between the person and the illness that has been ascribed to them (White, 1989). The traumatic event(s) associated with the crisis therefore come to define the person's identity, rather than being a life experience that he or she can relate to. The process whereby the person and those involved with him or her internalize the dominant societal discourses about mental illness has profound implications for their lives, as these internalized discourses 'have the effect of isolating persons from each other, and from the very contexts of their own lives. These discourses have provided for a way of speaking and thinking about life that erases context, that splits experience from the politics of local relationship' (White, 1993: 20).

Scott (1973a, 1991) argued that these cultural beliefs about mental illness create a powerful barrier to effective therapeutic intervention by severing the connections between the individual and the network of significant relationships which provide the context in which the crisis occurred, and by invoking the stereotypical notion of the mental patient as someone lacking in insight and personal agency.

CLOSURE

These dominant sociocultural beliefs about mental illness therefore exert a powerful influence on the life and relationships of the person who receives a psychiatric diagnosis. Scott uses the term 'closure' to describe this process in which a person in crisis can become disconnected from the network of intimate family and social relationships in which they ordinarily live their lives, and which provides the context for the difficulties which have occurred (Scott and Ashworth, 1967). Closure does not usually lead to family members abandoning one another in a physical sense, but rather a kind of dehumanizing process may follow. When a crisis is developing the family may be faced with an unbearable sense of hurt and pain. In the face of this, family members may cut off from the person who is regarded as ill. Scott and Ashworth (1967) argue that it is the bonds of love and affection which are severed, as it is these positive ties which are most painful. All of this begins to occur before the professional system is drawn into the situation, and psychiatric practice which fails to take account of the individual's social context may inadvertently exacerbate this rift:

> Closure can be a point of no return. A symptom . . . represents a partial death of that person as a social being. Being in the psychiatric space makes this death official. (Scott and Starr, 1981: 183)

Scott believed that once the invisible line is crossed which divides the 'mad' from the 'sane', this can be a point of no return. The person will always be viewed as 'ill', regardless of how 'well' they behave. Chronic psychiatric invalidism can be a kind of prison from which there is little prospect of escape or release, even for 'well' behaviour. Similarly, once the person has been defined as mentally ill they are in danger of finding themselves becoming further marginalized from the broader social world as a consequence of the stigma associated with psychiatric problems within our society (Goffman, 1963; Ramon, 1992).

CLOSURE AND PROFESSIONAL COMPLICITY

When a crisis occurs within a family, the beliefs of the individuals concerned may be in a state of flux (Caplan, 1964), and a number of commentators have argued that the intervention of professionals during this crucial time plays a major part in how the problem is subsequently viewed or defined within the family (Dallos *et al.*, 1997; Haley, 1980). When a situation becomes unbearably stressful for the members of a family or social group, a mental health professional may be invited into the situation to provide an 'expert' opinion. When this psychiatric interview leads to a diagnosis of mental illness being offered to a family member, then closure may ensue. Since the difficulties which the person is faced with are confirmed by the professional to be features of an illness over which the individual and their family have no influence or control, responsibility for managing the situation tends to be handed across to the professional system at this point.

The notion of the mental health professional as expert is particularly interesting in this context, as Scott (1973a) argues that prior to the professional being invited into the crisis situation, it has already been decided within the community that the person's conduct is a consequence of psychiatric disorder. The professional who is intervening in the crisis situation may therefore discover that their status as 'expert' is dependent upon their confirming this psychiatric account; an unwillingness to do so might lead to their opinion being discredited or considerable pressure being brought to bear to encourage the professional to intervene in the expected manner. Scott and his colleagues found from clinical experience that when these cultural beliefs about mental illness are challenged, then powerful reactionary forces may be mobilized in order to reassert the status quo.

As psychiatric nurses we are, of course, deeply involved in all of this, and the process of closure may touch our lives as well as the lives of our clients. Discussing the impact of closure on the professionals involved, Scott (1995: 6) comments:

> We become imprinted in the same manner that we have imprinted closure in the patient. This shows up in psychiatric practice where we are almost exclusively drawn to the negative, to what is wrong, and commonly fail to realize the primary importance of positive feeling. This is an imprint of the closed attitude. It runs throughout psychiatry.

A similar point is made powerfully by Deegan, who warns that when psychiatric professionals stop seeing patients as people, they become a bit less human themselves (Rosen, 1994).

One of the ways in which Scott proposed that professionals can avoid becoming complicit with the process of closure and the development of the treatment barrier is by refusing to talk with relatives or significant others about the client in the person's absence (Scott, 1973a, 1995). Secret talks of this nature are usually best avoided as they can easily reinforce the view of the client as unable to accept adult responsibilities or as lacking in 'insight'.

HOSPITALIZATION AS A FORM OF CLOSURE

When a severe crisis occurs in a person's life, a common professional response is to bring the person into hospital in order to try to contain the situation. The large majority of psychiatric admissions continue to occur on an unplanned basis in response to a perceived crisis or emergency (Moore, 1998). Closure can occur regardless of whether the person who is labelled 'ill' is treated in the community or in the hospital, but Scott suggests that hospitalization exacerbates the process of disconnection (Scott and Starr, 1981).

The importance of the concept of closure in relation to the experience of entering psychiatric hospital is supported by research undertaken by Whittle (1996), which examined the impact of admission on the causal beliefs of the people who were admitted, their families and the staff. This study suggests that following admission clients and their relatives became more attached to biological theories of causation, while psychosocial causal beliefs decreased significantly over the period of hospitalization.

Those clients who had been admitted previously also tended to be more strongly orientated towards a biological perspective. This change in beliefs did not seem to be influenced by the causal beliefs of the staff, who in this study were less strongly orientated towards biological beliefs. Whittle therefore suggests that this change in beliefs for clients and their families may have been linked with wider cultural assumptions about why people need to go into hospital, rather than occurring as a consequence of ideas presented to families by the staff. Whittle goes on to suggest a link between causal beliefs and treatment beliefs, in that clients who held biological causal beliefs were more likely to regard medication as the most relevant treatment for their difficulties. The perceived relevance of psychotherapeutic approaches generally, and family therapy in particular, seemed to diminish for these clients and their families.

Whittle also refers to previous studies which have suggested that when a person has been admitted to hospital once, he or she is more likely to request admission when experiencing subsequent life crises. Hospital admission as a response to a crisis situation therefore seems to be a particularly relevant factor in facilitating a process of closure in relation to interpersonal factors, and in the formation of a treatment barrier where family therapy is concerned.

CRISIS INTERVENTION

While the consequences of closure may be severe for the service user, their family, and also for the professionals who are involved in this process, Scott (1995) argues that crisis intervention provides an opportunity for professionals to actively intervene in order to prevent this occurring, rather than simply reacting to the situation in a more passive way. By visiting the person in their home setting as rapidly as possible, hospital admission can often be avoided. The resources of the family and the staff team can be drawn upon collaboratively in addressing the problems which led to the crisis, and decisions are made on the spot in the energy of the person's living situation (Scott, 1995). Scott also stresses the importance of involving the family or significant others from the outset (Scott and Starr, 1981). When this connection is established, even in those situations where hospital admission occurs, the family are more likely to remain actively involved in the therapeutic process as a consequences of their being included in the process from the outset.

Crisis intervention work based on Scott's ideas of closure and the treatment barrier reduced first time admissions by over 50 per cent (Ratna, cited in Johnstone, 1993; Scott, 1980). One of the features of this approach is the importance given by Scott to the quality of engagement between the professional and the person/family in crisis when contact is initially made (Scott, 1995). When entering into a situation of great tension the professional may feel pressurized into giving advice or making a treatment plan immediately. This feeling may be exacerbated for the professional by agency demands in terms of workload, efficiency and the importance of containing risk. However, Scott contends that a period of time spent with the service-user at the outset in which the professional allows her or himself to listen attentively and tune into the concerns of the person in crisis can save a great deal of time and money later, since it is the quality of the therapeutic relationship which is the most important factor in facilitating change (Andersen, 1997). Alternatively, the premature imposition of a treatment strategy is a recipe for future chronicity (Scott, 1995).

Within the field of psychiatry there has recently been a general resurgence of interest in the idea of crisis intervention teams, together with the related initiative of home treatment teams which can reduce reliance on hospital admission as a primary treatment strategy (Crompton, 1997; Riseborough, 1997). Based on research undertaken in Australia, Hoult and his colleagues have persuasively argued that intensive community treatment for people who are regarded as experiencing severe psychiatric problems can be more effective and cheaper than traditional hospital-based services, and seems to be preferred by people who access the service (Hoult *et al.*, 1984). Like Scott, Hoult (1993) argues that rapid, intensive help should be provided as early as possible in order to strengthen therapeutic alliances between the professional team, the identified client and his or her relatives, and also to help resume the person's normal routine as quickly as possible.

An important difference between the work of Scott and his colleagues and many of the more recently developed community models, however, is that those services developed in the 1980s and 1990s tend to be characterized by a strong allegiance to disease concepts of psychiatric disorder. Whereas Scott viewed early family-based intervention as an opportunity to prevent induction into a psychiatric career with the attendant processes of marginalization and stereotyping, more recent developments have tended to emphasize the importance of retaining a strong medical focus, for instance by advocating the use of psychoeducational approaches to family work which emphasize the importance of explaining theories of biochemical aetiology and medication compliance to families. The opportunities which crisis work may provide to undertake 'preventative' work, in the sense of avoiding the formation of a 'treatment barrier', is not featured to the same extent in more recent writings on the topic.[1]

An important exception is the work of Seikkula and his colleagues, working in the western Lapland area of Finland (Seikkula *et al.*, 1995). Mobile crisis intervention teams are the guiding principle of this team's service, and requests for psychiatric in-patient treatment are responded to by rapidly convening a meeting which includes the identified patient and those people who are closely involved with him or her as well as any professionals involved in the situation. All decisions about treatment are taken within these meetings, and are agreed through open dialogue between all participants. The development of this systemically orientated networking approach to crisis situations has led to a great reduction in the need to prescribe neuroleptic medication as well as admissions to hospital. Again, the full implications of this Finnish work are yet to be considered by purchasers and providers of services in the UK, perhaps because they require us to reconsider some long established beliefs about the treatment of schizophrenia – beliefs which are prevalent within the professional world and reinforced by perceptions about mental illness which are dominant in the society that commissions us.

CONCLUSION

The ideas of Scott and his colleagues continue to be of relevance and importance to mental health nurses and other psychiatric professionals. In recent years, issues such as underfunding of services and media coverage of community care 'failures' have led to increased public anxieties about people labelled mentally ill, and the levels and type of care they receive. Perceptions of the 'mentally ill' as irresponsible, dangerous and lacking in insight into their condition predominate in this context, and legislative initiatives have in turn been introduced which are aimed at increasing psychiatry's surveillance and monitoring roles in order to protect the general public. In other words, these are cautious times, and perhaps as a consequence, biochemical theories of psychiatric disorder have become strongly profiled, with an attendant emphasis on the importance of psychiatric diagnosis and compliance with medication. At the same time, however, the need to develop more effective and comprehensive community psychiatric services has led to a resurgence of interest in the idea of crisis intervention (Crompton, 1997; Riseborough, 1997).

This renewed interest in crisis services creates potential new opportunities for mental health nurses and other practitioners working within psychiatry. Opportunities, for instance, to understand and work with psychiatric problems within the social and interpersonal context in which they initially arose rather than simply view these problems as meaningless symptoms of an illness process; opportunities to work preventatively and reduce reliance on neuroleptics and hospital beds; opportunities to avoid colluding with the social processes which marginalize those people who have been designated 'mentally ill'. Nurses wishing to develop these opportunities will find encouragement and inspiration through returning to the writings of earlier innovators such as R.D. Scott and his colleagues.

ACKNOWLEDGEMENTS

I would like to thank Dr Chris Stevenson and Dr Dennis Scott for their helpful comments on previous drafts of this chapter.

NOTE

1 Within psychoeducational family therapy approaches there tends to be an emphasis on inducting the family into a medicalized understanding of the situation, thus potentially creating the conditions for closure to occur. Since it is likely, however, that the family will already be viewing the situation in illness terms, Scott (personal communication) proposes that a psychoeducational approach might provide a useful starting point for therapy when framed in a manner which both respects the current beliefs of the family while leaving an opening for different accounts to emerge.

REFERENCES

Andersen, T. (1997) Researching client–therapist relationships: a collaborative study for informing therapy. *Journal of Systemic Therapies,* **16**(2): 125–133.

Birch, J. (1991) Towards the restoration of traditional values in the psychiatry of schizophrenias. *Context,* No. 8 (Spring): 21–26.

Caplan, G. (1964) *An Approach to Community Mental Health.* London: Tavistock.

Clay, J. (1996) *R.D. Laing: a Divided Self.* London: Hodder & Stoughton.

Crompton, N. (1997) Early intervention begins at home. *Nursing Times,* **53**: 27–28.

Dallos, R., Neale, A. and Strouthos, M. (1997) Pathways to problems: the evolution of 'pathology'. *Journal of Family Therapy,* **19**(4): 369–400.

Goffman, E. (1963) *Stigma.* Harmondsworth: Penguin.

Haley, J. (1980) *Leaving Home.* New York: McGraw-Hill.

Hoult, J. (1993) Comprehensive services for the mentally ill. *Current Opinion in Psychiatry,* **6**: 238–245.

Hoult, J., Rosen, A. and Reynolds, I. (1984) Community orientated treatment compared to psychiatric hospital orientated treatment. *Social Science Medicine,* **18**(11): 1005–1010.

Johnstone, L. (1993) Letter to the Editor: Family therapy and adult mental illness. *Journal of Family Therapy,* **15**(4): 441–445.

Johnstone, L. (1994) Values in human services. *Care in Place,* **1**(1): 3–8.

Laing, R.D. (1967) *The Politics of Experience and the Bird of Paradise.* Harmondsworth: Penguin.

Moore, C. (1998) Admission to an acute psychiatric ward. *Nursing Times,* **94**(2): 58–59.

Parker, I., Georgace, E., Harper, D., McLaughlin, T. and Stowell-Smith, M. (1995) *Deconstructing Psychopathology.* London: Sage.

Ramon, S. (1992) Introduction: the concept of hospital closure in the Western world, or why now? In: S. Ramon (ed.), *Psychiatric Hospital Closure: Myths and Realities.* London: Chapman and Hall.

Riseborough, S. (1997) Home but not alone. *Nursing Times,* **93**(52): 23–25.

Rosen, A. (1994) 100% Mabo: de-colonizing people with mental illness and their families. *Australian and New Zealand Journal of Family Therapy*, **15**(3): 128–142.

Scott, R.D. (1973a) The treatment barrier: Part 1. *British Journal of Medical Psychology*, **46**: 45–55.

Scott, R.D. (1973b) The treatment barrier: Part 2. *British Journal of Medical Psychology*, **46**: 56–67.

Scott, R.D. (1980) A family orientated service to the London Borough of Barnet. *Health Trends*, **12**: 65–68.

Scott, R.D. (1991) Family relationships and outcome in schizophrenia focusing the often unperceived role of the patient. In: N.R. Punukollu (ed.), *Recent Advances in Crisis Intervention*. Huddersfield: Institute of Crisis Intervention and Community Psychiatry Publications.

Scott, R.D. (1995) *The Barnet Crisis Service*. Paper delivered at the 25th anniversary meeting of the Barnet Crisis Service.

Scott, R.D. and Ashworth, P.L. (1967) 'Closure' at the first schizophrenic breakdown: a family study. *British Journal of Medical Psychology*, **40**: 109–145.

Scott, R.D. and Ashworth, P.L. (1969) The shadow of the ancestor: a historical factor in the transmission of schizophrenia. *British Journal of Medical Psychology*, **42**: 13–32.

Scott, R.D. and Starr, I. (1981) A 24-hour family orientated psychiatric and crisis service. *Journal of Family Therapy*, **3**: 177–186.

Seikkula, J., Aaltonen, J., Alakare, B., Haarakangas, K., Keranen, J. and Sutela, M. (1995) Treating psychosis by means of open dialogue. In: S. Friedman (ed.), *The Reflecting Team in Action: Collaborative Practice in Family Therapy*. New York: Guilford.

Warner, L., Ford, R. and Holmshaw, J. (1997) Don't just role over and die. *Nursing Times*, **93**(52): 30–31.

White, M. (1989) The externalizing of the problem and the re-authoring of lives and relationships. *Selected Papers*. Adelaide: Dulwich Centre Publications.

White, M. (1993) The politics of therapy: an interview with Michael White by Lesley Allen. *Human Systems*, **4**(1): 19–32.

Whittle, P. (1996) Causal beliefs and acute psychiatric hospital admission. *British Journal of Medical Psychology*, **69**: 355–370.

Introduction to Chapter 12

Gary Winship

by Phil Barker

Gary Winship is representative of a new generation of young British psychiatric nurses who have retained their sense of history, and use that history to help them frame their future, and that of their chosen discipline. Gary Winship presently works as a nurse psychotherapist in the Psychotherapy Services in West Berkshire. He is, however, a 'Maudsley-trained' nurse, and has – perhaps appropriately – brought much of that part of his own personal and professional history with him to his present work. Gary also is involved in the preparation of other nurses, to become clinical nurse specialists in psychotherapy, and has been one of the key people involved in the development of a national interest group in psychoanalytic psychotherapy. That said, he does not restrict himself to any specific domain of therapy. He is, perhaps, interested in 'learning from patients' as his chapter will reveal. Although he is widely educated, his conversation is, invariably, simple and straightforward. He has come to appreciate the value and significance of true 'conversation' and hones this as, perhaps, his primary therapeutic tool.

In this chapter, Gary steps back from his specific area of interest – therapy and therapeutic environments – and addresses some of the wider, contextual factors within which therapeutic environments might be embedded. He offers a challenge to much of the orthodoxy of the past twenty-five years and is not afraid to own his own uncertainties about the world of care, and his own difficulties in judging the 'need for care'.

In this chapter, Gary Winship offers some sobering, simple, yet we believe inherently wise observations about the context of care, and the value of asylum as part of our social world. He is an optimistic man. We presume that this will endear him to patients as much as colleagues. Yet, he does not allow his optimism to rule him, and he is conscious of the nature of the challenge posed by the immediate future, where political power appears steady, and the need to cater for the dispossessed of society may be the lowest of all vote-catchers.

12

The birth of the *new* asylum?

Gary Winship

BRIEF

Mass decantation from psychiatric institutions has been the pre-dominant feature of mid- to late twentieth century psychiatry. Dissolv-ing the old psychiatric asylum system was thought to be the answer to the age-old problem of treating the mentally infirm. However, the highly published shortcomings of 'community care' suggest that the ethos of de-institutionalization towards a psychiatry without walls may have been over-determined in its aspirations. Rather than successful integration of the mentally ill in the community we appear to have entered an era of fragmentation characterized by increased fear in the general public's mind and new levels of social exclusion of psychiatric patients.

The 'Mental Health Reference Group' established by the Health Secretary (1998) has been charged with developing a system of care in the community which will include the deployment of 'mini asylums' in the community. That we may have de-centred prematurely from the old asylum system is debatable, though the resurgence of interest in creating (or re-creating) a new version of the asylum in the form of a mini asylum suggests we may have underestimated the containing function of the asylum institution. *We are compelled to re-appraise the very concept of the asylum.* The task of creating a new dimension of a localized or mini asylum might offer a window of opportunity for creating a better version of asylum, though it would be pure folly to forge ahead without a rigorous re-appraisal of the dimensions of containment offered by the old system; that which was good and that which was not good. In the therapeutic community tradition of psychoanalytic enquiry into institutional process, I attempt to locate a good enough psychiatry in the history of the asylum system before offering an inchoate schema for considering *the therapeutic principles of asylum and its dimensions of containment.*

INCLUDED OUT

Foucault's (1961) study *Madness and Civilization* suggests that since the Middle Ages social forces have incited a concertina-like phenomenon whereby the willingness to gather in madness has been countered by a force of ejection. The violence, theft and other anti-social activities of the homeless lunatics on the streets of Paris during the twelfth and thirteenth centuries led to the creation of the first *l'hôpital* for the insane. The authorities felt that it would be economically wise to contain the mentally infirm by housing them in one place and thus the hospital was created. The dangerousness of the insane had confounded the charitable and religious organizations and thus, for the first time in the history of medicine, the insane were rounded up and locked away.

Foucault contrasted this early example of confinement with the banishment to the countryside of the mentally ill during the 1400s. Locked out of the city gates, the homeless and the vagabond mad folk were excluded from the church as well as charity and were instead expelled to the high seas on an imaginary journey to reason on the *ship of fools*. Foucault argued that the banishment of those perceived mentally infirm was born out of a belief that somehow reason would rule if only madness were out of sight. Foucault further charts the journey through the next centuries where 'treatment' was again characterized by a re-gathering with patients being imprisoned and manacled, whipped and once again treated as criminals. This period of imprisonment was again followed by further exclusion to the countryside, this time in the shape of the out-of-town asylums which were ascendant from the late nineteenth century onwards.

The overall impression that one gets from Foucault's study is that organized psychiatric treatment has oscillated through the ages between imprisonment and banishment. Either way, psychiatry has always been an instrument of inhumanity and torture up to and including modern times. Even the radical work of Tuke at the Retreat in York with the development of moral treatment is critically scrutinized. Foucault sees Tuke as replacing the idea of punishment with the invocation of guilt and the need for sober repentance in the face of a wrathful god. The great period of incarceration is superseded by moral confinement.

Foucault assigns the emergence of psychiatry to the domain of the irrational where reason is suspended consistently and surpassed by the general folly of mankind. His is an unremitting anti-psychiatry stance and though his critique may have been one among several major catalysts for progress, alongside Goffman for instance, we should be wary to damn psychiatry in its entirety based on Foucault's reading alone of a complex discourse.

David Russell's (1997) study of the history of treating the mentally ill, *Scenes From Bedlam*, is something of an antidote to Foucault. Written from the inside of psychiatry as a practitioner, Russell provides a sympathetic appraisal of a more often blighted profession. Russell's book was one part of the 750th anniversary celebrations of the joint Bethlem and Maudsley Hospital, first established in 1247 as the Priory of St Mary of Bethlehem in Spitalfields, London. The Maudsley celebrated its '750 years keeping mental health in mind' (as their celebration slogan read) with a corporate memoir and several events, including a special exhibition at the Museum of London with paintings by Richard Dadd and Louis Wain among others on loan from the Tate Gallery and the Bethlem archive, photographs of patients showing 'mal humour' from the late 1800s, several antiquated devices for restraining patients and the two giant statues of 'Raving madness' and 'Melancholia', sculpted by Caius Gabriel Cibber [b.1630], which were originally situated at the entrance of the Bethlem at Moorfields from 1676–1815 (now the Imperial War Museum) were exhibited too.

Despite these prestigious celebrations there were dissenting voices (in the *Guardian* and *Nursing Times*) arguing that there was little cause to celebrate the longevity of the Bethlem; rather its *continuing* history was cause for public outcry. David Russell's (1997) meticulously researched book, emerged as contrary to popular opinion as a sympathetic text. The result of his several years of trawling through the archives of the Bethlem is one of the most incisive, lucid and exposing historical accounts of treating the mentally ill to date. Packed with previously unpublished data, photographs, eye witness accounts and a particular emphasis on the work and accounts of the non-medical staff of the asylum, Russell's work ranks alongside Foucault (1961) and Scull (1979) as an essential text in mapping the emerging history of psychiatry.

Russell's findings depart from Foucault and Scull insofar as he highlights that the treatment of the mentally infirm has more often than not been underpinned by a well-intended philanthropy, particularly from the mid 1800s onwards following the liberating work of Tuke in York and Pinel at Bicetre. Even in the darkest times of manacled patients, wet sheeting and whipping, psychiatry was not alone in its punitive attempts at curing madness. Russell cites the writings of Sir Thomas More, an esteemed Christian visionary known for his humanity, who decreed that a deranged member of his congregation, known to be an ex-patient of Bethlem, should be whipped and ejected from his church. Russell presents a persuasive case that psychiatry has been no more guilty than being of its time.

Even the 'darker ages' would seem to be unfairly enshrined in Hogarth's famous painting of Bedlam in the mid 1700s, *The Rake's Progress*. When one delves deeper into Hogarth's famous sketch of

Bedlam, viewing it in the context of the other several sketches that depict the caddish Thomas Rakewell's demise through his sloth, prostitution and gambling, we discover that the scene from Bedlam is more like a moral aphorism than accurate documentary. Hogarth's sketch may be contrasted with other commentaries. For instance, Charles Dickens visited the Bethlem in the late 1850s and found much to praise in the work of the senior physician Charles Hood, who had helped the hospital to adopt a more humane and caring approach following an inquiry and subsequent damning report from Lunacy Commissioners in 1851 (cf. Russell, 1997). Dickens wrote; 'The light has been let into Bethlem: it gives light of the flowers on the wards: it sets the birds singing in their aviaries: it brightens up the pictures on the walls ... the quickness and completeness of change made by a reversal of old superstitions on the treatment of insanity ... The star of Bethlem shines out at last' (cited in Russell, 1997: 152). A few years later, Sheppard, a prominent politician, was even more ecstatic about the treatment of the mentally ill:

> I will venture to say that there is no class of person better cared for in the United Kingdom than the insane. The best sites in the Kingdom are selected for their palaces. The fat kine of our fields are stored for them, clothing of the warmest and supervision of the best are provided for them. They are rained upon by sympathy ... and fenced about with every sort of protection which legislature can devise. Magistrates, guardians, commissioners, friends inspect them, visit them, record their grievances, register their scratches, encourage their complaints, tabulate their ailments. (Sheppard [1872] quoted by Russell [1997])

Though Sheppard's assertions may be over-enthusiastic, the transformation from the human warehouse of Bedlam into an aspiring good-enough mental hospital was sure and steady. The twentieth century saw an increasing humanitarianism underpinning psychiatry with interventions becoming palpably less and less invasive. The proliferation of the use of talking cures (cf. Aubrey Lewis, 1934) and the widening net of drug therapy saw an ever greater eradication of deep insulin therapy and psychosurgery.

CLOSING THE ASYLUM

Yet despite the progress that was been made in transforming many large psychiatric hospitals into thriving therapeutic communities with radical new therapeutic approaches, the image of the psychiatric hospital as a 'bin' emerged during the twentieth century and remained an unshiftable indictment. Most people would still associate psychiatry with the infamous institution portrayed in the film *One Flew Over the Cuckoo's Nest* (1972) rather than the more benign image presented in Vincente

Minnelli's film *The Cobweb* (1952), based on the psychoanalytic model of treatment at places like the Chestnut Lodge Sanatorium in the USA.

The backdrop to the mounting antagonism towards the psychiatric asylum included Goffman's (1961) damning profile of one institution which became enshrined in the public and political psyche. The hierarchical structure of the asylum and its oppressive social system and organization had caused Goffman (1961) much concern following his observation study of a Washington psychiatric institution during the late 1950s. Likening what he called *the tinkering trades* of medical psychiatry to the repair work provided by other people in the service of the public, Goffman noted how the axiom of the respected customer in psychiatry was not apparent in the hospital hierarchy. Goffman's noted that at best the patient was maligned and bullied and at worst grossly maltreated. Patients and staff tended to 'conceive of each other in terms of hostile stereotypes, staff often seeing inmates as bitter, secretive and untrustworthy, while inmates saw staff as condescending, high-handed and mean' (1961: 18). The communication was such that Goffman felt that staff could not hear patients unless they were shouting.

At the same time as Goffman's American study there was increasing public antipathy towards the asylum system in the United Kingdom. In the same year that Goffman published his study, in a now famous speech, Enoch Powell (1961) signalled the death knell for the Victorian asylums: 'There they stand, isolated, majestic, imperious, brooded over by the gigantic water tower and chimney combined, rising unmistakable and daunting out of the countryside – the asylums which our forefathers built with such immense solidity.' It was this 'solidity' that Powell saw his way to deconstructing. He argued that a new model of community care would mean that the need for hospital beds would be halved over the following fifteen years. This was a theoretical impetus which, gathering momentum during the late 1960s, gave rise to innovative district and community services firstly in Croydon and then Manchester (Bennett, 1991).

In 1975 a crucial government document, *Better Services for the Mentally Ill*, recommended that psychotic patients be treated in general hospitals rather than in the old specialized hospitals. Thus, the asylum was assigned to the chopping block and by 1983 its fate was sealed in the Griffith Report; the schedule for closure was finally delivered in the 1991 *Health of the Nation* document, which promulgated the shutting down of the ninety remaining mental hospitals by the year 2000. Until 1983 over 95 per cent of psychiatric beds were in institutions and by 1995 the number of psychiatric beds had decreased to less than half with an increasing number of patients being treated in day hospital and by community health care teams (Bennett, 1996; Rogers and Pilgrim, 1996).

There were only a few voices which challenged this ideology during the 1970s and 1980s and brief rearguard action against closures was fought by only a few clinicians. The South East Thames Regional Health Authority, in conjunction with its regional nursing advisory committee, did produce a document in 1986 called *The Need for a Haven* which posited that the mental hospital had a positive role in the future treatment of psychiatric illness in cases where patients needed refuge or haven away from their immediate surroundings. But this document was barely a whisper in the high winds of change. The closure roller-coaster was too far down the track for turning back.

Why there was such silence about the closure of psychiatric hospitals is worth considering. After all, the furore raised by the public when it is mooted that a general hospital is to be closed is usually considerable. So why should there be such unresponsiveness regarding the psychiatric hospital suggests that quite different forces are at play. Perhaps the demise of the psychiatric asylum is another incarnation of what Foucault describes as a wish to deny the existence of madness, the rejection of the need for asylum amplifies an idea that psychiatric services are of no use, in this way the general public may perpetuate the illusion that there is no such thing as madness.

Politically, the closure of asylums was a scheme borne out of a number of disparate trends rather than one coherent philosophy according to Barham (1992). In his study Barham argued that; 'far from returning home after a long period of exile, many people with mental illness are being ejected from the refuges that had protected them from the brunt of market forces' (1992: 99). Barham asserted that the idea of providing opportunities for patients to self determine their lives was in fact little more than rhetoric disguising the 'dumping of a group of people whom it has become too costly to maintain in the old welfare style' (p. 99).

The momentum of closing psychiatric hospitals has rather eschewed the fact that many asylums have come to operate in ways very different to the institutions that Goffmann (1961) portrayed. Indeed, the psychiatric system, as it has emerged out of the old asylum system, has been moving towards ever-greater degrees of democracy and enfranchisement over the past fifty years. It could be said that the thrust towards community care and the idea of treating mentally ill patients in their own homes may deprive the mentally ill patient of a chance of 'retreat' to the refuge of the countryside. Whereas once banishment to the 'bin-on-the-hill' might have instilled fear, today admission to a countryside asylum for a time of recuperation from the trauma or breakdown might seem a desirable treatment choice.

While Foucault observed the casting out of the mentally ill into the countryside meant banishment to an inhospitable wasteland of wandering isolation, life beyond the city now has a bourgeois air. The inner city is the common place of paranoid congestion, whereas the countryside now is the rich domain of replenishment, leisure, clean air and rejuvenation (Hinshelwood, 1993). Does it seem like such an ill-founded idea to suggest that some patients might well fare much better recovering in the countryside rather than in hectic and cramped inner city psychiatric day hospitals? If so, we might think of the demise of the asylum as a corrupted political act whereby the poor are excluded from access to the richness of the countryside.

So what is the bequest of the psychiatric asylum? The progress of psychiatry may have been slow but when charted within the context of a wider social perspective, for instance the tardy demise of slavery, or the drawn out history of capital punishment, the treatment of patients in psychiatry seems to have a fairly benign track record by comparison. There may have been much to live down in the twentieth century, such as the radical biological attempts at cure – like ECT, brain surgery and drugs – but in time to come even these methods might be considered of their time. When faced with the extremities of the human condition like psychosis, mania or melancholia, to reach for idiosyncratic attempts at cure has some rationale.

It is not quite a case of 750 years of hurt and shame and now psychiatry is coming home, but in the grand scheme of history it is perhaps possible to talk about the liberation of the mentally ill as we near the end of the millennium. The asylum has been the melting pot where radical progress has been made. Today no practitioner, even a neurologist would deny the fundamental value of talking therapy or being kind and caring towards a patient. Freud's dream that his talking cure would inherit the promised land of psychiatry has perhaps been realized. Even given the many conflicts arising out of radically different therapeutic approaches, including the continued dominance of the biomedical model, humanity reigns throughout for the most part. The psychiatric patient is ever more enfranchised.

INSTITUTIONAL NEEDS?

Jeremy Holmes (1992) has argued that the idea of 'psychiatry without walls' suggests a progressive transformation towards a post-institutional agenda. But enthusiasm for the grand scheme of embracing the mentally ill in the community-at-large needs to be tempered. Indeed, we might wonder whether the rejection of the idea of institutional care has been well judged. The demise of the ideology of 'care in the community', both in the public and professional mind, suggests that as a model, community care has elemental problems in practice.

The idea of a mini asylum, based in the community, offers a bridge between the two previous paradigms of countryside institutional care and non-institutional community care. An experimental alternative system of combining hospital care with community care was established in the 1970s at the Maudsley Hospital in London. The innovative unit was called the District Services Centre (DSC). The idea for the DSC arose largely out of the research of Wing, Brown *et al.* and their 'Camberwell Studies'. They identified a need to develop local services for patients in the catchment area who were otherwise sent some thirty miles away to be treated at Cane Hill Hospital in Surrey. As a local psychiatric hospital, the DSC established a trail-blazing day support unit for hundreds of patients, with on-site residential facilities (twenty beds) for acute episodes. Thus, the model of short-term or respite in-patient care aimed to maximize the patient's independence. Although the centre was built on the main Maudsley site it was free-standing, away from the main ward blocks with its own separate entrance.

Over a period of several years from the early 1980s I came to know the DSC as a centre of unshifting psychiatric chronicity, itself an institutional revolving door. The residential section of the unit endured the highest levels of violence in the joint Bethlem and Maudsley hospitals and the atmosphere of the centre was characterized by staff fatigue and stress. In the day hospital patients would lounge about in huge wafts of cigarette smoke, indolent, medicated, with barely enough life energy to scrounge their next cigarette from passers-by. Those who were considered more capable engaged in what was well described as 'industrial therapy', monotonous tasks such as packing boxes which enabled some patients to earn small amounts of money. The industrial therapy offered a type of false or pseudo-maturity, that somehow these needy patients were normalized; going to work.

The goodwill efforts of the staff were palpable, but within an ethos bereft of therapy efforts seemed futile in the face of such chronicity. Morale was always low, with high staff turnover and during the time I spent there, apart from risking lung cancer, I learned something of how tall an order it was to sustain a model of a positive local treatment with very complex patients. Even though there were efforts to negotiate between patients and staff, setting goals and so forth, the problem lay in an inherent shortfall in the culture that refused to acknowledge the *in-depth* therapeutic needs of the patient group.

The task of empowering patients is complex. Although the acutely disturbed patient may be approached as an equal, empirically in practice the authority may need to rest with the staff. For instance a patient who wants to kill themselves or others is necessarily disempowered by the clinical decision of the carers. Jonathon Pedder (1991) has well described 'the fear of dependency in therapeutic relationships' that underpins much of psychiatric practice. He argues that in the West there is a belief that dependency is bad and that independence is good. The denial of dependency would seem to be an apposite notion when it comes to thinking about the DSC. It was as if the culture of the place was one where there was a refusal to look at how needy the patients were. It seemed to me that the level of acting-out was directly proportionate to the unacknowledged dependency needs. I recall one patient who would regularly take to lying down in the middle of the road in front of the building. She would be admitted and then would be discharged again quickly.

By no means would I argue that the rest of the Maudsley Hospital was getting it right when the DSC was struggling so. But elsewhere there were lower levels of violence, lower levels of re-admission and fewer enforced on-site sections. To my mind, the DSC in its short-term efforts to keep patients in their homes ultimately failed the patients it was treating in the long term.

The asylum system was so often criticized as an instrument of what became referred to as 'the nanny state', that is to say, the welfare system that was perceived as being soft and too nurturing, making it too comfortable for patients. The philosophy of the DSC came to represent a project that attempted to maximize independence in order to throw off the idea of the 'asylum as nanny'. In order to counter this idea the welfare system became a place where harder, tougher decisions were made. Short, sharp shock treatments for young offenders were recommended and a pervasive air of fear evolved where treatment design attempted to offer *social containment through deterrence.*

Is it possible for us to re-appraise this erstwhile welfare ideology by developing a model of care which manages to transcend the divide of promoting individual blame on the one hand and accepting the dependency needs of the patient on the other? Is it conceivable to create a humane psychiatric system which acknowledges patients in-depth needs without the system being charged with infantilizing collusion?

DIMENSIONS OF ASYLUM

Our attempts at operating without asylum have faltered so we must begin with an acknowledgement that illness limits patients, in varying degrees, to levels of reliance on others. This reliance on others might be considered as *an institutional need for asylum.* That is to say, patients in acute stages of psychological illness overtly or inadvertently express a need for a safe haven. We need to be better prepared to grapple with the dependency or attachment needs that so confound psychiatry. Community care has suffered from a lack of centredness and the absence of the solidarity offered by the asylum. The sturdy image that is brought to mind with the old asylum may be one similar to Enoch Powell's description of the water towers of our forefathers. We might be well prompted to consider recapturing the inherited object constancy that the asylum represented.

After years of embedded denigration of the concept of asylum, I suggest that we need to deconstruct our understanding of what 'asylum' signifies. When we refer to 'political asylum' the image conjured up is one of safety and haven away from oppression. The notion of 'psychiatric asylum' stirs up quite oppositional visions of cold incarceration, banishment and shackled impoverishment. The asylum in the public mind has become a negative social interface for the collision of internal disturbance and the external world. That is to say, the asylum has been the container into which a wide range of fantasies are projected. We have possibly underestimated the function of the asylum in containing anxiety not only within that of the patients but also without, insofar as it has become a receptacle for public projection; venomously attacked and vilified with our fears of mental illness.

A radical shift in mindset is needed if we are to more positively appraise the concept of asylum. It would otherwise be *impotent to broach the idea of creating a mini asylum without an optimistic construction of the potential of such an institution.* On this point I find myself at odds with Isobel Menzies-Lyth's fascinating, though essentially pessimistic outlook on institutions. At the end of her career studying a multitude of settings, including the fire department, the hospital and the nursery among others, she concludes: 'Unfortunately, I have come to a depressing conclusion: that institutions have a natural tendency to become bad models for identification' (Menzies-Lyth, 1988: p. 42). She further argues that the larger the institution the greater the likelihood of the institution becoming a bad model of identification.

I have so far offered an alternative rendering of her depressing diagnosis *vis-à-vis* the psychiatric institution, in particular with a reading of David Russell's (1997) affirmative contribution to the history of psychiatry. Based on this reading, I would argue that psychiatric institutions have overall been enclaves of humanizing progress. Contrary to Menzies-Lyth, I would argue that psychiatric institutions have an innate tendency towards being good models of identification and the larger the institution the greater likelihood of good identification (two examples that come to mind are Parliament and the NHS). As I described earlier, psychiatry has a comparably benign historical track record as a civilizing institution compared to other pathways of humanitarian progress such as the abolishment of slavery and capital punishment.

If we are to rescue back the positive connotations or values of asylum, we need to challenge the traditions of Foucault, Goffmann and Menzies-Lyth. Is it possible to re-frame the notion of psychiatric security which brings to mind punitive policing, keys and locked doors and instead think about security as the benign force that counters insecurity. Can we talk about 'secure attachment' rather than security, thus opening the way for a discourse of therapy that brings to mind theories of benign attachment and holding (Adshead, 1998)? If we make a conceptual shift such as this, the idea of security becomes both legitimate and necessary. Likewise, can we reclaim the necessity of containment which currently bears the hue of hostile incarceration, instead, can we think of containment as a process whereby disturbed patients can experience being held, both physically and in mind.

I suggest we need to consider *the therapeutic principles of asylum*, as if they are needed by some patients. Containment and security are so often patient-determined. Our efforts to empower patients are often met by an equal and opposite force which perpetuates the patient in a needy role. For example, I saw several drug-addicted clients in Lewes prison, all of whom suffered from underlying disturbances which were symptomatized by their addiction to drugs. One of the clients was very clear as to the reason why he put scaffolding through the window of a large department store in Brighton; he said he felt unsafe and wanted to be in a secure place that was warm.

To my mind if we are to help patients be 'without' a psychiatric institution we need to understand what being inside the institution means to them. In considering the dimensions of containment offered by the asylum system I propose to use Henri Rey's notion of the 'asylum as brick mother' as a starting point (Rey, 1975; cited in: Holmes, 1992). In humanizing the asylum, Rey's metaphor draws our attention to the psychodynamics of the function of asylum. I suggest that the containing function of the asylum can be sub-divided into four dimensions or psychic envelopes. I think about these in terms of containing skins.

Dimension 1: the outer skin

Under this heading we think about the physical boundaries – fences, walls and doors – which enact the organizational processes that culminate in the structure of the asylum as a space away from other spaces. We might think about the body of the asylum in terms of 'exoskeleton', the outside layer that frames and protects the patient inside, keeping the outside world as separate.

The relationship between the asylum and the local community enjoins far more osmotic forces of engagement than is usually given credence. In the realms of the space and location of containment, the implications for the closure of the 'local asylum' community are often forgotten (there is a paucity of sociological research in this area). For instance many psychiatric hospitals have been integral to the life of local village communities. The physicality of the asylum with its water tower as it broods over the local village is only one aspect of the juxtaposition of the hospital and the local community lifeworlds. The asylum and its patients in many areas became part of the local way of life, arguably replenishing local village businesses and so forth. It is possible that the exoskeleton of the asylum needs visibility (something which is worth considering with the creation of the mini asylum). Attempts to camouflage the asylum smack of an apology-creating facade of integration extending the doomed strain of likeness and denying the indubitable fission of difference. All of us need to have a club, society or work place where we enjoy membership and affiliation. The disenfranchised psychiatric patient also needs a locus of belonging. In this way membership of the visible psychiatric institution is a transitional phenomenon.

Dimension 2: skin on skin

The body of the patient may be actually held inside the asylum, historically by tools of restraint and more recently by the hands of the staff. The history of the strait-jackets, wet blankets, manacles and other accoutrements is relevant here and the transition of these procedures as the means of control, discipline and punishment to more therapeutic 'holding' techniques is notable in the evolution of this dimension. These are the occasions when skin-on-skin contact between staff (most commonly nurses) and patient includes the physiognomy of restraint. A memory of physical containment lies at the heart of the need for physical containment. A patient may need to be embraced or forcibly held. The physical holding may be part of the process whereby the bodily ego of the psychotic patient is re-established (Winship, 1998).

The process of restraint by the clinical staff includes the use of chemical and psychological interventions (the talking therapies). However, how aware current practitioners are of the significance and meaning of the process of physical restraint will be worth considering. Arguably the recent development in the use of *control and restraint*, a psychiatric procedure derived from police force, returns psychiatry to a more punitive practice.

Dimension 3: social skin

This includes the lifeworld network of the patient's peer relations and the everyday events of routine structures in the milieu. The intensity of these peer relationships and structures may vary. For instance, a patient may be contained by attending a day programme or an out-patient group on only one occasion each week. At the other end of the spectrum of intensity of containment is the social system that surrounds a patient who may be receiving 24-hour care as an in-patient. The structures of the milieu and influencing organizational systems including the people who work within the system including the secretarial, ancillary support staff, domestics, cooks, engineers and so forth, all contribute towards a social containment of the patient. This dimension has been a focus of a great deal of interest in this country in the form of the therapeutic community movement and in the USA in the milieu movement.

Dimension 4: an inner skin

The patient's internal world and his capacity to hold or contain himself is the final dimension of containment – it has something of the potential of 'asylum in mind' that makes rehabilitation or re-integration possible. Where the internal psychic skin cannot hold, the patient retreats from the cluastrom of his social connectedness. The process of reconnecting with others during the course of therapy is a prerequisite to a successful rehabilitation where the development of an internal asylum (in mind) may act as an object constant necessary to the recovery and re-integration of the patient in society.

SUMMARY

The total treatment environment is based around the recognition of the intertwining psychic and social forces which are necessary to bond people together, helping them in their healing and ultimately sustaining their recovery. It was once the work of the Therapeutic Community movement from the 1940s onwards to transform the old asylum system into the type of institution where all parts of the community worked together for the general good. To a great extent this work remains unsurpassed and might well be the basis for creating the infrastructure of the 'new asylum system'. It is towards the task of extrapolating the psychodynamic infrastructure of the asylum that I have provisionally developed a 'quadripartite model' to describe the levels of physical and psychical containment offered by the asylum system.

REFERENCES

Adshead, G. (1998) Personal communication.

Barham, P. (1992) *Closing the Asylum. The Mental Patient in Modern Society.* Harmondsworth: Penguin.

Bennett, D. (1991) The drive towards the community. In: G.E. Berrios and H. Gaskell Freeman (eds), *150 Years of British Psychiatry: 1841–1991*. London: Royal College of Psychiatrists, pp. 321–332.

Foulkes, S. H. (1938) Review of Uber den Prozess der Zivilization by Norbert Elias. *International Journal of Psycho-Analysis*, **19**: 263.

Foulkes, S. (1948) *Introduction to Group Analytic Psychotherapy.* London: Heinemann.

Foucault, M. (1961/1989) *Madness and Civilization*. London: Routledge.

Goffman, E. (1961/1968) *Asylums*. Harmondsworth: Penguin.

Hinshelwood, R D (1993) The countryside. *British Journal of Psychotherapy,* **10**(2): 202–210.

Holmes, J. (1992) Psychiatry without walls. Some psychotherapeutic reflections. *Psychoanalytic Psychotherapy,* **6**(1): 1–12.

Lewis, A. (1934) Melancholia: A Historical Review, reprinted in *The State of Psychiatry* (1967). London: Routledge.

Menzies-Lyth, I. (1989) *The Dynamics of the Social,* vol. II. London: Free Association Books.

Pedder, J. (1991) The fear of dependence in therapeutic relationships. *British Journal of Medical Psychology,* **64**: 117–126.

Powell, E. (1961) Opening Speech at Annual Conference. London: National Association for Mental Health.

Russell, D. (1997) *Scenes From Bedlam.* London: Balliere Tindall.

Scull, A. (1979) *Museums of Madness.* London: Allen Lane.

Shepard, E. (1872) On some of the modern teachings of psychiatry. *Journal of Mental Science,* **17**: 499–514

Thonicroft, G. (1998) Care in the community. *Guardian,* 11 February 1998, p. 9.

Winship, G. (1995) Democracy in psychiatric settings: individualism versus collectivism. *Therapeutic Communities,* **17**(1): 31–45.

Winship, G. (1998) Intensive care psychiatric nursing. *Journal of Psychiatric and Mental Health Nursing,* **5**: 1–5.

POSTSCRIPT: A REFLECTION ON CHARITY AND ITS DISCONTENTS

On my way to work each morning I pass by a modern church, slightly set back from the road in a residential suburb of Reading. One autumn morning I happened upon a fracas outside the church. A smart middle-aged woman was firmly ushering an old woman down the path away from the glass doors of the church. The old woman was carrying a cumbersome load of several bags she appeared reluctant to leave. Even though I was a distance away, the old woman's disconsolate mutterances were audible; you f--ing this and that, I could hear her saying. By the time I reached the church the old woman was on the pavement and the usher was returning towards the church. The old woman seemed unsure of where to turn next and stood looking absently around her. She did not notice me as I passed by. She continued conversing with herself in a stream of cusses. My brief proximity to her evoked in me the feeling of alienation I have experienced when close by a floridly psychotic patient hearing voices. What could I do? I walked on to work and noticed as I looked back that the church woman had returned to pruning the bushes by the path.

I have an association. Once I tried to help an old lady across the busy Anerley Hill Road in South London near the junction of Maple Road. It was 1983 and I had just moved into the area so did not know the locality very well. The old woman was tiny, old and bent and appeared to be stranded on the bollard island in the middle of the road. She was much less than five feet, her face was leathery and crumpled and I guessed that she was at least seventy years old. She was looking at the cars and lorries whizzing up and down in the quickening pace of early rush hour. I crossed to the middle of the road and said, 'Do you want to get to the other side?'. She didn't respond and instead she continued watching the traffic. Sure that she was frozen with fear I took her by the elbow and nursed her across the road. She was agitated but I took this to be a measure of her fear so remaining firm to my task we made a reluctant passage to the other side. She offered me no thanks and instead, much to my chagrin, she turned around and walked back onto the central island, re-assuming her original traffic watching position. I later discovered that she was well known to locals for her strange but regular past-time. Over a period of several years I would happen upon her in the middle of the road on many occasions.

If there is a moral here it is something about the clumsiness of measuring need. The old bag lady was clearly in need of help, disenfranchised, cold and agitated. She was treated most uncharitably. The old lady that I tried to help was not in need of my help and my charity was unnecessary. The case of the Holloway vicar (1996) who let a disturbed schizophrenic into his church to make him a cup of tea only to end up being stabbed in the back is only one case in point of the cost of misjudging the needs of the patient and forcing premature empowerment. Such events are emblematic of the potential disarray when it comes to relying on church and charity in containing the wanderings of the mentally infirm.

When I was on call as the duty nurse in charge of a large London teaching hospital one evening I was hastened to an acute unit because a patient was disturbed and threatening, refusing to take his medication. When I arrived I found the young man in his room talking incoherently to himself as if responding to hallucinated voices. He had been unresponsive to the staff and when I spoke to him he did not seem to hear me. I noted that his bed did not have a sheet on it. There were faeces on his covers and smeared on the wall. The staff told me that he was 'on a programme of disattendance for his acting out'. They did not know what to do. I asked the staff to bring fresh bedding which they did and without further ado I began to change his sheets and re-make his bed. After a short while the patient began to help me. We pulled his bed out from the wall and put a mattress cover on and cleared the excrement. He calmed, became more responsive and a short while later took his medication.

This was a young staff team who had misunderstood the needs of the patient and whose expectations of self care were premature. The team were operating within a culture which had not grasped that relationship between autonomy and authority involved a transition from regressive needy states through progressive levels of maturity. The patient's mental state in this case was such that he required a greater degree of nursing intervention than he was receiving. I am not proposing unsolicited succour. Donald Winnicott's clinic motto 'We should first of all ask, not what we can do, but rather what little needs to be done!', seems apposite, but what a patient sometimes needs is an acceptance of their primary dependency needs.

Introduction to Chapter 13

Jeffrey Fortuna

by Phil Barker

Although various authors have addressed, at least in passing, the social and cultural significance of mental illness in this text, much of that discourse has been 'Western', framed by modernism or post-modernism. We are aware also, that despite the assumption that mental health care is largely about *care*, there has been no specific consideration of this vital human construct. In particular, we are aware that much of our concerns about power and authority involve what we *do not like* or in some way seek to *reject*. In Jeff Fortuna's work we find an example of what many people might well be seeking as an alternative: a consideration and exploration of compassion, and its contribution to the whole care and recovery process.

Jeff Fortuna is the Director of the Windhorse Project in Northampton, Massachusetts where, along with his wife Molly Fortuna, and a team of therapists, 'housemates', family members and friends, he leads a programme of recovery for people in psychosis. The Northampton project is merely the latest stage in a 20-year journey for Jeff Fortuna and his colleagues, seeking to establish a genuine sense of community, based on acceptance, respect and compassion. The Windhorse programme grew out of the theoretical and practical work of Ed Podvoll, with whom Jeff worked, and much of Jeff's orientation to people in great human distress or difficulty stems from Podvoll's work. However, Jeff Fortuna has also made his own, special and important, contribution to the literature on recovery – a contribution that reflects clearly his experience at the 'care-face'.

There are clear lines of linkage between the Windhorse Project and Loren Mosher's Soteria House, and Ronnie Laing's Kingsley Hall. Apart from anything else, all express an appreciation of the importance of the history of therapeutic communities. The nature of the community that is Windhorse, and which is so eloquently described by Jeff Fortuna, is, however, at least one stage on from those original 'human home' projects.

The importance of interconnectedness and belonging, and the importance of the simple tasks of everyday living, spring from his chapter. When we visited Windhorse last year, Jeff and his colleagues gave so freely of their time that we felt as if we had always known him; and perhaps in the sense that he explicates here, we had.

13

Therapeutic households

Jeffrey Fortuna

> If somebody is dancing in the sky and breathing air, that is worse than if he is sitting on the earth, eating dirt – which has more potential. It's as simple as that! (Chogyam Trungpa, 1983: 10)

It is refreshing to encounter a clinical intervention, in the vast array of modern psychotherapeutics, that is simple, effective, has withstood the test of time, and is grounded in common sense. 'Therapeutic households' is one such refreshing situation. Therapeutic households, as 'domestic ground,' is the experience of earthy practicality that is the literal basis of human life. As 'domestic discipline,' it is the practice of working with the elemental details of ordinary life situations with attentive respect. As 'domestic harmony,' it is the establishment of an open healing environment that supports wholesome human relatedness. This precise care of domestic ecology encompasses the lives of everyone involved in the treatment of and recovery from mental disturbance, and is the cornerstone of any flourishing community or culture.

The impulse to provide household treatment for disturbed persons has manifested historically in a variety of forms. The Geel Community in Belgium (Parry-Jones, 1981), founded in 1480, demonstrates the large-scale effectiveness of this social arrangement. At its height, the Geel Community successfully cared for 15,000 mentally ill people within the local, rural community.

Bruno Bettleheim, the world's foremost authority on the treatment of autism, wrote the following description of his own experience:

> From 1932 until March 1938 (the invasion of Austria) I had living with me one, and for a few years two, autistic children. To make this a therapeutic experience for them, many conditions of life in our home had to be adjusted to their needs. This was my initial experience with trying to create a very special environment that might undo emotional isolation in a child and build up personality. (1967: 8)

Ex-mental patients have advocated for this kind of treatment for as many as 150 years (Perceval, 1961), and it appears to be generally appreciated as a commonsensical idea. However, most attempts to create therapeutic households have lacked the theoretical views, skilful means and practices needed to accomplish this intention.

In modern Western treatment, the mentally ill are often grouped together or hospitalized in in-patient settings, transitional halfway houses, long-term group residences, cooperative apartments, lodge programmes, rural environments, crisis centres, nursing homes, and board-and-care homes (Lamb, 1984). This treatment pattern carries several liabilities: it fosters a chronically mentally ill life-style based on diagnostic stigma; it creates a medical-psychiatric establishment with the potential to abuse power (Perceval, 1961; Foucault, 1965); and it compounds the effects of mental illness by creating settings in which patients' psychopathologies overlap. 'Highly disturbed people, when grouped together, run the risk of becoming more confused; when they are in the company of healthy people, they are likely to become more healthy' (Podvoll, 1985).

With the failure of deinstitutionalization and increasingly inadequate funding, the problem of providing decent housing and residential treatment for the mentally ill is acute. The result of this unmet challenge is clear: 'Depriving the chronic patient of food, shelter, and clothing, thus subjecting him to the vicissitudes of the elements, undoubtedly contributes to his deterioration and repeated decompensations' (Lamb, 1984: 157). This situation is reaching the proportions of a national emergency and requires resourceful innovation in order for positive change to occur (Pollack, 1977). It is within the context of this urgency that the following model of therapeutic households is presented.

My intention in writing this article is to elaborate on the principles of the specialized treatment households described by Edward Podvoll (1985) in his presentation of Maitri Psychological Services (MPS). MPS is a comprehensive treatment service that provides individually tailored care for psychologically disturbed persons. The three interrelated components of this service are:

1 therapeutic households, which are established as the locus of treatment;
2 basic attendance provided by team therapists; and
3 intensive individual psychotherapy provided by a primary therapist.

To isolate one of these components for the sake of discussion could be misleading to the reader because all three interact to form a total environment. The MPS approach departs from mainstream psychiatry in avoiding the grouping together of disturbed persons in one facility.

Instead, each MPS patient lives with two housemate-therapists in an ordinary household setting in the local community. This situation is similar to a foster care arrangement.

This chapter is addressed to concerned professionals, mentally disturbed persons, and friends and family members of the mentally ill who are faced with domestic chaos and confusion. This chapter can be used as a practical guide or 'recipe' of environmental healing principles. These principles are applicable to the households of *both patients and therapists*.

THE ADMISSION PROCESS: MUTUAL INTERVIEWING

A prospective patient enters the MPS programme through a process of mutual interviewing during which everyone gets to know one another. The applicant and his family members meet with the MPS senior clinical staff to explore the potential patient's current problems, aspirations and intentions, as well as what MPS can offer to him. The applicant meets with several team therapists for three hours at a time to sample a variety of activities and relationships, and to articulate personal interests, talents and disciplines. In addition, the potential patient consults individually with the primary therapist to discuss the interplay of health and illness in his personal history and to briefly experience the interpersonal openness that is the basis of intensive psychotherapy (Podvoll, 1985). The applicant visits several existing treatment households to candidly discuss the MPS programme with patients and room-mates. This discussion can range from the level of housework to the unravelling of complex delusions. These meetings with current patients and/or past patients – 'graduates' – of the MPS programme are especially poignant; they often include the sharing of personal hopes and fears, stories of failures in other treatment settings, and glimmers of enthusiasm about the recovery of a meaningful life. This experience contrasts with the often dire diagnostic predictions of medical specialists – for example, that one is destined to a life of chronic psychosis. The applicant's family members are encouraged to participate fully in these discussions.

The overall tone of the interview pattern is one of candour, inquisitiveness and genuine human contact. This thorough interview process, lasting several days, is necessary in order to elucidate the nature of the MPS programme and to discover a mutual working basis. An essential component of this working basis is an active interest on the part of the clinicians, the potential patient, and the patient's family in making a personal commitment to the work: we do not accept patients against their will. If the proper conditions exist, a six-month commitment to the programme is requested of the patient and family. Our experience has shown that this amount of time is necessary in order for the patient to settle into the therapeutic household and new interpersonal relationships. Several months are needed in order to ascertain whether or not the patient is making significant progress through the stages of recovery (Podvoll, 1985). As well, this commitment allows sufficient time for the patient's family to contribute their own sanity into the programme by helping to set up the patient's household and permitting the treatment team to share in their understanding and appreciation of the patient.

DOMESTIC GROUND: EARTHY PRACTICALITY

- *Establish the household: involve the patient in a collaborative effort to create a decent, simple, and cheerful place to live.*

Rather than admit the patient to a pre-existing facility, the MPS staff, along with the patient, work to create a fresh household environment. This is in itself the beginning of treatment. Initially, a team leader and a team of therapists are selected to join the primary therapist in working with the new patient. Then, individual and group meetings are scheduled. The group's primary task is to find two housemates, one female and one male, and a suitable house to rent. This may be the first time the patient has helped to establish a home and find housemates. The patient's family members are encouraged to remain in town for two weeks to facilitate the patient's difficult adjustment to a new place and new people. In the beginning, patients may fear that they will be unable to cope with the many details that demand their attention in this new setting. However, with the support of the MPS team these intimidating tasks become opportunities for resourcefulness. All of our patients have surprised themselves in this regard. They are always more capable than they had anticipated and all of them have felt the grounding and strengthening effects of these practical beginnings. The experience of the MPS staff is that this phase of collaborative treatment is important in setting a tone of mutual respect and cooperation.

- *Pay deliberate attention to details: emphasize an earthy simplicity in arranging the domestic environment. Domestic details become the 'pull of gravity' or antidote to mental wandering.*

The patient confronts real choices. For instance, what kind of house does he prefer and in which part of town? What colours, what window sizes, and how much light does he prefer? Will pets be allowed in the household? Does he want a garden to cultivate or a yard to care for? Confronted with these details, the patient's ordinary, but perhaps atrophied, sense perceptions, discrimination and concentration begin to awaken. This increasing alertness moves the patient beyond painful self-preoccupation, confusion and the cloudy hangover of previous institutional life. One patient described this process as follows:

> For me, this raised some interest in the outer world, for example, making decisions on the basis of what would I like? how do I want to live? This was in contrast to the flat, institutional environment I came from, in which I had no ability or right to exert myself [in] this way – a very simple, practical, and, thus, refreshing task.

Chogyam Trungpa emphasized the importance of this mundane approach:

> Try to work with the pinpoint of the situation by being very practical and ordinary. Working with environment basically means bringing people down to earth. If a person suddenly loses his gravity and floats up to the moon, he wants to come back to earth. He may be willing to become sane. At that point, you can teach him something. He will be so thankful to feel the gravity on the earth. You can use that logic in every situation. Earth is good. (1983: 10)

Repeatedly bringing attention back to the immediate situation is a powerful antidote to the desynchronization of mind, body and environment that originally fostered the mental disturbance (Podvoll, 1980). The patient is gently guided to apply these 'contemplative' efforts in order to ground himself in the here-and-now.

● *Create open communication: cultivate a style of honest interaction between the patient and his housemates to encourage 'maitri' or gentle precision.*

The process of interviewing potential housemates accompanies the house search. Successful applicants must have a sane and orderly approach to their own household, practise a contemplative discipline, and have an overall allegiance to self-development or personal journey in all aspects of their life. Integrity and a sense of humour are considered invaluable assets. Generally, such applicants are as dedicated to learning as they are to earning a living. The patient and the team leader interview applicants, once again in the spirit of discovering a mutual working basis. When one housemate is selected, he or she joins the interview team. The thorough precision of establishing the household may be experienced as mundane, tiresome, or boring by the patient or housemates, especially in contrast to the 'life and death' issues that have brought the patient into treatment. One patient stated that: '[I] already know all about housekeeping. In fact, my mother was a perfectionist around the house and, in teaching me everything she knew, contributed to my obsessiveness. What I really need to figure out is the meaning of life and then to decide if I should bother with a clean home at all.' The challenge is to discover a sense of profundity, in relation to the household and to establish the working basis of a 'domestic discipline'.

Much of the MPS approach is based on the Shambhala tradition. Chogyam Trungpa described two central themes of the Shambhala tradition – the 'heaven principle' and the 'earth principle' – as follows:

> Traditionally, heaven is the realm of the gods, the most sacred space. So, symbolically, the principle of heaven represents any lofty ideal or experience of vastness and sacredness. The grandeur and vision of heaven are what inspire human greatness and creativity. Earth, on the other hand, symbolizes practicality and receptivity. It is the ground that supports and promotes human life. Earth may seem solid and stubborn, but earth can he penetrated and worked on. Earth can he cultivated. The proper relationship between heaven and earth is what makes the earth principle pliable. (1984: 129–30)

So, for example, the MPS view or theory that complete recovery from psychosis is possible (Podvoll, 1985) is an aspect of the heaven principle, whereas organizing and maintaining a household budget and ledger is in the realm of the earth principle. When properly joined, the heaven and earth principles result in the experience of being grounded and demonstrate the profound meaning of householding in human life.

In an MPS household the domestic ground is established with these principles in mind. First the house is rented and furnished, the patient and housemates move in, and food is purchased. Then increasingly familiar sights, sounds and odours permeate the atmosphere. The patient settles into his new relationships with the team therapists and individual psychotherapist. The patient's and housemates' participation in proper exercise, adequate sleep patterns and regular eating habits are gently attended to. A housewarming is held to mark the establishment of the new household. Guests include the entire MPS community, close friends and the patient's family. These gatherings are often joyous and ignite a spirit of celebration.

DOMESTIC DISCIPLINE: BACK TO BASICS WITH ATTENTIVE RESPECT

● *Establish a schedule: shared household meals, chores, and, especially, regular house meetings foster continuous sensitivity toward the well-being of the entire situation and accentuate the contrast between daydreaming and perceiving reality.*

The daily schedule begins to bring order to the activities of the MPS household residents. It becomes a crucial reference point which sharpens the residents' awareness of the boundaries of experience – for example, the boundaries between work and relaxation. House meetings are attended by the patient, the two housemates, and the team leader; they are held weekly at the MPS residence These meetings serve as the central forum for managing household matters. For instance, chores which are shared equally and rotated among the household members, are assigned during these meetings. At least three meals are scheduled each week to be attended by all the house members; each member is scheduled to take a turn preparing the communal meal. The purchasing, preparation, serving and clean-up of meals are discussed thoroughly. Initially, the dinner atmosphere may feel formal and strained, which may reflect a carry-over of tension from mealtime situations with the patient's family of origin, but it soon relaxes into an atmosphere of enjoyment. Hosting dinner guests becomes an opportunity to refine social graces and to extend generosity. Often team therapists participate in the cooking, dining and housework in order to further enliven the household.

During the house meeting, the group frequently focuses on the quality of the relationships evolving among all the household members and, thereby, avoids excessive preoccupation with the patient. Some meetings begin with a 'check-in' about how each resident's week has been or about current personal concerns that might impinge on the household atmosphere. The professional boundaries between the patient and housemates are openly discussed in these meetings rather than being unilaterally established. The patient is also encouraged to give feedback to his housemates concerning the fulfilment of their job responsibilities. For example, the patient might comment if one of his housemates is spending inadequate quality time at home due to social distractions or work outside of the household. In fact, the housemates' daily lives are an important source of vicarious learning and inspiration for the patient, although they may also engender a temporary depressive impoverishment in the patient if the contrast between the quality of his own life and the lives of the housemates is too great. However, the sharpness of this contrast can awaken further discrimination. The inevitable boredoms, irritations and complaints that arise when people live together are ventilated in this atmosphere of honest communication. This may be an imposing challenge for a patient who has been previously isolated due to painful self-preoccupation with illness.

Honest, reciprocal communication between the patient, the housemates and the other team members is the basis of consensus decision-making and is at the foundation of the MPS therapeutic community. This kind of communication expresses our conviction that truth, itself, is medicine; that truth can heal. Chogyam Trungpa wrote:

> The main point is to tell the truth to your patients. Then they will respond to you, because there is power in telling the truth rather than bending your

logic to fit their neurosis. Truth always works. There always has to be basic honesty; that is the source of trust. When someone sees that you are telling the truth, then they will realize further that you are saying something worthwhile and trustworthy. It always works. There are no special tips on how to trick people into sanity by not telling the truth. (1983: 7)

In such an open social system (Jones, 1982), the patient has the opportunity to foster the personal and professional development of the staff members and, thereby, exercise his innate compassionate impulses. The frustration of these compassionate impulses is itself a source of mental illness (Searles, 1979b). In this sense, the household is maintained for the benefit of everyone. This phenomenon of 'mutual recovery' of staff members and the patient is the bedrock of any healing community.

Mutual recovery can be both a refreshing and confusing experience. The patient, as the person who is designated as ill, may want to relax into being cared for: having a maintenance crew to clean his house, having his meals prepared, or simply remaining in bed, and all the while secretly resenting being 'baby-sat'. These regressive tendencies are highlighted by the demands and attractions of ordinary daily life. R.D. Laing relates the story of a deeply regressed woman who, after several years of withdrawal at the Kingsley Hall community (Berke, 1980), actually got up from her bed of faeces when she smelled the aroma of a delicious soup (personal communication, 1986). The patient's perception of contrast leads to a choice of whether to allow himself to slip back into the shadows of delusion or to face the bright world that surrounds him. Through this choice, the patient may begin to recontact a sense of appreciation and responsibility.

In turn, the MPS housemates may begin to wonder if they are therapists, friends, or, perhaps, even patients themselves! Not only are their personal domestic lives fully exposed to the patient and other team members, but their professional lives are also open to view and completely supervised. Regressive tendencies on the part of the house-mates – such as treating the patient as if he is damaged, dependent, or like a child – are viewed as defensive. This kind of distancing serves to maintain a rigid sense of the housemates' role security and to ward off the threat of insanity – that is, both the patient's and the housemates' own insanity.

The difficulty of openly sharing the same environment and, literally, breathing the same air with a patient in an acute or residual phase of mental disturbance has been unanimously attested to by the MPS housemates. At the same time, 'breathing the same air' is actually the common ground of healing. The housemates are in the ideal situation to experience this because they maintain a 24-hour-a-day involvement with the patient's household. Chogyam Trungpa wrote:

If you and the other person are both open, some kind of dialogue can take place which is not forced. Communication occurs naturally because both are in the same situation. If the patient feels terrible, the healer picks up that sense of wretchedness: for a moment he feels more or less the same, as if he himself were sick. For a moment the two are not separate and a sense of authenticity takes place. From the patient's point of view, that is precisely what is needed: someone acknowledges his existence and the fact that he needs help very badly. Someone actually sees through his sickness. The healing process can then begin to take place in the patient's state of being, because he realizes that someone has communicated with him completely. There has been a mutual glimpse of common ground. (1985: 7)

In the context of such a direct relationship, the patient and the housemates are free to explore the true meanings of friendship and healing – questions that concern all of us regardless of mental illness. One may wonder whether such complete openness leads to wild, group indecency or whether the intimacy becomes too claustrophobic for the patient. One might wonder about the professional boundaries and ethics involved in the situation. Ongoing contemplative practice, training in compassion, and clinical supervision serve to maintain the housemates' awareness of their inner experience and the outer situation in the household. Good manners and basic human decorum follow naturally. The purity of the clinical intention is maintained when the patient's best interests are kept in mind. This is not to deny that strong emotions may occur among the residents, but these emotions can be worked with honestly.

An MPS programme 'graduate' addressed this issue as follows:

I think no matter how hard you try there will be a wall, there will be a distinction between therapist and client. It will be the 'us and them' mentality, definite boundaries . . . There [is] a definite barrier in the codes of professional ethics. Those walls are real, that's all I can say.

In contrast, a housemate described his experience this way after five months' work:

I felt more relaxation within the formality of dinner. It was no longer just flat. I began to wonder: Who's providing what medicine for whom? for whose needs? mine? the patient's? I feel it's so good for me . . . There's some dissolving of roles as we first thought of them . . . more fluidity of responsibility . . . more emptiness of roles, particularly of my healing someone. It feels so ordinary, three people living together, living their lives. There's more uncertainty about my role.

This particular experience was reported during a formal clinical presentation to a supervision group of housemates and team leaders.

Presentations of this kind are detailed descriptions of specific domestic situations, which include the housemate's own experiential process. The supervisory discussion may focus on the housemate's well-being, his relationship with the other housemate or the patient, or simply the general decorum of the household. Gatherings such as these are important supportive components of the MPS community fabric.

● *Encourage a contemplative attitude: cultivate recurring awareness of the basics of daily life. The MPS staff is brave enough to step beyond therapeutic aggression and the patient is brave enough to step beyond the nightmare of self-preoccupation. The techniques recommended for cultivating awareness are, for example, simply sitting together quietly for several minutes before a housemeeting.*

As the treatment evolves, regressive tendencies that lead to illness and professional ambition erode and honest communication and precision with domestic details gather strength. Trustworthy kindness that can accommodate potential chaos pervades the household. This is what is meant by the term *maitri*, or loving kindness:

> The basic point is to evoke some gentleness, some kindness, some basic goodness, some contact. When we set up an environment for people to be treated, it should be a wholesome environmental situation. A very disturbed or withdrawn patient might not respond right away – it might take a long time. But if a general sense of loving kindness is communicated, then eventually there can be a cracking of the cast-iron quality of neurosis: it can be worked with. This can be arduous. But it is possible, definitely possible. (Trungpa, 1983: 9–10)

The actual means by which a wholesome situation can be created involve bringing compassionate discipline to the elemental conditions of the household, such as money, food and shelter.

This is a worthy challenge for the 'warrior-healer'. 'Warrior,' in this sense, has nothing to do with aggressive treatment of an enemy – of a disease syndrome – rather it means to overcome aggression itself. Aggression is the tendency to hold oneself intact in order to ward off any genuine contact with the situation at hand. Chogyam Trungpa defines a warrior as 'one who is brave ... The fundamental aspect of bravery is being without deception' (1984: 108). A 'healer' is simply someone who attends to another person's recovery of intrinsic health. A 'warrior-healer', then, is a person who joins bravery and compassionate attentiveness.

One subtle form of therapeutic aggression that is inevitably faced in any treatment programme concerns overly conceptualizing or psychologizing about the patient's alleged illness. For example, the therapist may pigeonhole a patient in a diagnostic category, or regard temporary mental disturbance as a chronic, fundamentally destructive suffering, but may ignore the history of sanity (Podvoll, 1983). The result is that the therapist thinks of himself as a rescuer or saviour, but is actually a self-righteous 'dedicated physician' (Searles, 1979a). My own experience of this subtle therapeutic aggression is described in the following excerpt from a journal I kept during an eight-month period as an MPS housemate:

> I am in the middle of working with domestic irritation/anger/aggression and my tendency to distance from S [the patient] *is* aggression. I point out to him that he is crazy in these ways and he responds, 'You don't understand! This is real and spiritual!' I try to put S in his place as the patient and myself in my proper place as the bastion of sanity to keep myself intact? The more fixed ideas I have about myself or S the less fresh air and ventilation there is in the environment.

The therapist begins to feel a certain arrogance and political dominance in this situation, which can lead to endless abuse of power. The therapist's attitude can influence his perceptions and clinical action and become self-reinforcing. This attitude leaves little breathing room for the natural unfolding of the patient's process of recovery of the basic state of health temporarily obscured by mental disturbance. The practice of the warrior-healer is to step beyond this therapeutic aggression into a genuine relationship with the entire situation. This is the personal practice of all the MPS team members but, in particular, of the housemates, because their lives are so embedded in the therapeutic household. The understanding and adoption of this practice is one of the objectives of the Master's Program in Contemplative Psychotherapy at The Naropa Institute. That objective is stated as follows in *The Naropa Institute Institutional Self-Study Report* (1986): 'To teach students to recognize that there is no difference between personal and professional integrity and that an essential part of being a psychotherapist is to manifest health in one's personal life.' Essentially, this means to regard all the different areas of one's life – personal, social, professional, spiritual – as a common training ground for developing awareness and compassion. To relate to the rugged elements and vicissitudes of daily life in this way is to adhere to 'domestic discipline'. Chogyam Trungpa affirmed this:

> Enlightened society must rest on a good foundation. The nowness of your family situation is that foundation. From it, you can expand. By regarding your home as sacred, you can enter into domestic situations with awareness and delight, rather than feeling that you are subjecting yourself to chaos. It may seem that washing dishes and cooking dinner are completely mundane activities, but if you apply awareness in any situation, then you

are training your whole being so that you will be able to open yourself further, rather than narrowing your existence. ... Shambhala vision is based on living on this earth, the real earth, the earth that grows crops, the earth that nurtures your existence. (1984: 97)

- *Strengthening maitri: appreciation of increasingly clear sense perceptions grows in the domestic setting. A gentle, truthful approach to human intimacy causes truth to become medicine for bewilderment.*

In order to meet the 'meditation-in-action' challenge described in the previous section, MPS has utilized mindfulness-awareness meditation. In this meditation practice, one assumes an upright posture and places one's attention on the breath. The discipline trains one to bring one's wandering attention back from daydream to awareness of the immediate environment. The patient is offered instruction in mindfulness-awareness meditation at an opportune point – either when the patient has requested instruction or when the staff believe it would be appropriate. It is important to note that the essence of the meditation practice has already permeated the MPS household setting through the continual reminders by the team therapists to synchronize mind, body and environment in ordinary activity. The intent is to awaken the patient's mind through his sense perceptions and to establish an appreciation of the actual situation at hand. This sheds light on the true meaning of the ubiquitous folk saying, 'Come to your senses!' This contemplative approach has been especially useful when withdrawing patients from psychiatric medications; it provides an alternative means by which to clear and stabilize the patient's attention.

It is this contemplative approach that sets a tone of gentle precision in the MPS household and in the entire treatment setting. Further domestic learning occurs because situational and interpersonal feedback is more clearly perceived by the residents and simple cause-and-effect situations become obvious. For example, food preparation, serving, eating and clean-up skills become naturally refined and appreciated when household members pay more attention to them. Household meals become celebratory gatherings to which everyone contributes. The entire household situation becomes nourishment, in the larger sense, by supporting the residents' basic health and personal growth. The patient begins to make friends with the experience of being at home in his body on this earth. This experience is in poignant contrast to the common psychotic suspicion, 'Maybe I'm from another planet.' For instance, one patient stated, on entering the MPS programme, that one of his main goals was to create and maintain a household and to learn to live with others after years of 'solitary mind sailing'. He has now accomplished that goal.

DOMESTIC HARMONY: CRISIS AND RELAXATION

● *Host the circle of friends: radiation of hospitality is essential, whether in welcoming guests to household meals or in hosting the attendants of a disturbed house member. Expand the virtue of the household through the practice of compassion.*

The term *domestic harmony* is prone to unrealistic interpretations. One might think it means creating a heaven-on-earth to achieve domestic bliss. To another the term might mean maintaining 'walled in security' from the hostile, demanding world of the workplace. To a third person, domestic harmony may imply a licence to establish a kingdom of personal territory, as in the expression 'a man's home is his castle'.

From the point of view of environmental treatment, domestic harmony means maintaining a decent, organized household that welcomes and supports wholesome activity. As Chogyam Trungpa stated, the goal is to:

[create] harmony in your environment in order to encourage awareness and attention to detail. In that way, your physical environment promotes your discipline of warriorship. Beyond that, how you organize your physical space should be based on your concern for others, sharing your world by creating an accommodating environment. The point is not to make a self-conscious statement about yourself, but to make your world available to others. When that begins to happen, then it is possible that something else will come along as well. That is, when you express gentleness and precision in your environment, then real brilliance and power can descend onto that situation. If you try to manufacture that presence out of your own ego, it will never happen. You cannot own the power and magic of the world. It is always available, but it does not belong to anyone. (1984: 110)

It may seem unwise to speak of 'power' and 'magic' in the treatment of psychosis because that disorder often involves the megalomanic abuse of personal power (Podvoll, 1983). For instance, domestic violence erupts within the privacy of the home: personal power can be abused on one's home turf according to one's own law. The central issue is aggressive territoriality – of experience, or of the household. The challenge to the warrior-healer is to create and maintain a healing environment that is in harmony with the natural laws of the Shambhalian earth principle. The MPS approach contrasts with the common Western therapeutic model, which is based on a rigid hierarchy, one-way observation and communication, and the mystique of medical power. In the latter approach, authentic human intimacy may become a technical intervention, rather than a spontaneous occurrence.

When an MPS household is settled – that is, when respect for natural boundaries that promote basic health has been established – a 'circle of friends' may be properly hosted. 'Circle' implies containment and fluid communication; 'friend' means someone who genuinely cares. In this case, the circle includes the MPS treatment team, friends and families of the patient and housemates, and members of other MPS households. In a larger sense, this circle of friends is analogous to any gathering of people who attend to the welfare of a sick person in their community. It is common knowledge that along with the dissolution of the extended family or clan in our Western society, the mental health industry has formed to provide human services. In spite of the community mental health movement, however, the mentally ill have been relegated to a lower class on the cultural fringe. Through the creation of a contemplative healing community, which regards the disturbed person as a valued member, MPS works to recover the folk wisdom of the extended family.

● *Accommodate order and chaos equally: a housemate in crisis is neither complained about, punished, nor excessively indulged. Appreciate the complementary nature of health and illness.*

Sometimes an MPS household enters a state of crisis. Perhaps the patient has become increasingly despondent and suicidal or is forcing a psychotic transformation that may culminate in transgressive actions that are dangerous or 'beyond the law' (Podvoll, 1983). With the mounting intensity, the team's attention focuses on the household as well as on the patient. Under these circumstances, the household is kept especially neat and fresh. Plenty of aromatic, nutritious food is prepared. Fresh flowers are often arranged. The housemates are relieved of some responsibilities so that they are better able to process the personal strain and frustration that develop from 'breathing the same air' with the patient. Clinical supervision is provided more often in order to ventilate the feeling of claustrophobia and to strengthen the team's precision. An atmosphere of combined caring and alert accommodation prevails; the patient is not punished or humiliated by the staff for his 'inappropriate' behaviour. Speech is used skilfully to comfort the patient and to reflect back the simple cause-and-effect relationship of the patient's or team members' confused interactions. Protective measures can be taken if necessary, such as confiscating flammable materials, alcohol, car keys, or sharp objects. These measures protect the safety of the environment and minimize the patient's possible negative actions and their consequences; they are not intended as an attempt to dominate the patient's extreme state of mind. Major tranquillizers can be used to slow down the speed of the patient's thought process without obscuring his natural consciousness and, thereby, allow the interpersonal situation to relax.

The psychological intention of the team members is even more significant during a time of crisis because a highly disturbed person perceives with exceptional accuracy. Hypocrisy, fear, deception and conflict among the team members can only serve to provoke further paranoia and acting out in the patient. For example, cycles of escalating aggression between staff and patients are commonly observed in traditional hospital settings.

Sometimes crises are resolved easily and other times with more difficulty; there is no magical antidote. In the MPS approach, the team practices its warrior discipline; it strives to maintain authentic, healing friendships with everyone involved and to give precise, loving care to the patient. The situation in an MPS household in crisis is analogous to the situation in any household where a member is physically ill or has been injured. All of the family members or housemates are deeply affected. The issue is how the household members and community gather together to help.

Sometimes a person has to be allowed to be sick without making too big a mess. Recovery is not a linear process but an organic development of wakefulness, which requires patience with the interplay of health and illness. The team and the patient learn to persevere despite the highs and lows. In any case, it is only common sense to create a wholesome environment in which to care for someone who is ill.

● *Develop the patient's proper relationship to space: cultivate a sense of genuine presence in physical and interpersonal space by skilfully synchronizing mind, body and environment. Remain grounded on the earth with attentive respect.*

A central symptom of mental illness is the disturbance of spatial relations (Chapman, 1966). This disturbance can occur in any spatial sphere: in the orientation of one's body in physical space; in communicating with others in interpersonal space; or in relating to the space of one's own imagination and projection. In *Hidden Dimension*, Edward Hall wrote: 'Man's feeling about being properly oriented in space runs deep. Such knowledge is intimately linked to survival and sanity. To be disoriented in space is to be psychotic' (1969: 105).

In order to allow the patient to explore and develop spatial relations, MPS has utilized a technique based on Buddhist psychology, called *maitri space awareness practice*. This meditation practice involves lying in a particular bodily posture in one of five differently coloured and shaped rooms while maintaining experiential awareness. Although the technique involved in this practice and its clinical effectiveness require further explanation, such an explanation is not within the scope of this chapter. However, we have found that the carryover to one's daily life is increased appreciation of the senses and attentiveness to full-bodied presence in physical and social space. Chogyam Trungpa wrote:

> To communicate skilfully a person must be aware of interpersonal distance – a sense of whether he should reach out or wait. That kind of distance becomes very distorted so that communication is handled unskilfully; and there is frustration about that blindness. This brings on aggression and the demand for pain. ... Because one becomes completely overwhelmed, involved, self-centred into so much *here* one loses the distance. That is the extreme of egocentricity.
>
> It seems that setting up a certain kind of general situation for the person is more effective [than using encounter-group or analytical methods]. One starts with the basic physical situation of food and living environment. The whole idea of using the situation is to communicate with the unbalanced person so as to awaken him, so you start on the basic level of survival, the instinctive level, the level of the animal realm. The person should have some feeling of instinctive simple communication. Start that way. Then having established that kind of simple communication on the level of survival the rest become much easier and quite obvious. (1978: 71–2)
>
> The outcome of domestic harmony is the patient's development of a proper relationship with the varieties of space that promote health. These include the physical and social space of the household as well as the open psychological space that can accommodate order and chaos, or health and illness. To protect this harmony, furnishings, interpersonal encounters and concepts are simplified. The MPS housemates share a household with the patient, which is neither withdrawn from nor continuously engaged in therapeutic work. An almost palpable atmosphere of relaxation, precision and hospitality develops in the domestic setting. This is often obvious to members of the housemates' families, who are encouraged to reside in the household during visits. It is this domestic harmony that hosts the circle of friends, and the wider MPS contemplative healing community. In this way, the patient is provided with an interesting and expansive healing environment in which the complexities of chaotic mental disturbance can naturally unwind.

CONCLUSION

The key point made here is that an appreciation of the sanity and goodness of the earth principle can be embodied in a therapeutic household. It is the ground, discipline and harmony of a healing environment. Respect for and attention to the ordinary details of domestic life are a powerful antidote to mental disturbance, the root cause of which is the wandering of mind from environmental details. The MPS approach establishes the domestic environment as the cornerstone of a sane world. Future research in environmental treatment could begin with simply taking a fresh look at our own household.

If we apply the perspective of heaven, earth and man to the situation of the world today, we begin to see that there is a connection between the social and the natural, or environmental, problems that we are facing. . . . Human beings destroy their ecology at the same time that they destroy one another. From that perspective, healing our society goes hand-in-hand with healing our personal, elemental connection with the phenomenal world. (Trungpa, 1984: 130, 132)

SUMMARY: HOW TO ESTABLISH A THERAPEUTIC HOUSEHOLD

1 Domestic ground: earthy practicality
   - Establish the household
   - Pay deliberate attention to details
   - Create open communication
2 Domestic discipline: back to basics with attentive respect
   - Establish a schedule
   - Encourage a contemplative attitude
   - Strengthen maitri
3 Domestic harmony: crisis and relaxation
   - Host the circle of friends
   - Accommodate order and chaos equally
   - Develop the patient's proper relationship to space

REFERENCES

Berke, J.H. (1980) Therapeutic Community Models: II. Kingsley Hall. In: E. Jansen (ed.), *The Therapeutic Community.* London: Croom Helm.

Bettleheim, B. (1967) *The Empty Fortress.* New York: Free Press.

Chapman, J. (1966) The early symptoms of schizophrenia. *British Journal of Psychiatry,* **112**: 225–251.

Foucault, M. (1965) *Madness and Civilization, A History of Insanity in the Age of Reason.* New York: Pantheon.

Hall, E.T. (1969) *Hidden Dimension.* New York: Doubleday.

Jones, M. (1982) *The Process of Change: From a Close to an Open System in a Mental Hospital.* Boston, MA: Routledge and Kegan Paul.

Laing, R.D. (1986) Personal communication.

Lamb, R.H. (ed.) (1984) *The Homeless Mentally Ill.* Washington, DC: American Psychiatric Press.

Naropa Institute (1986) *Institutional Self Study Report. Submitted to the North Central Association of Colleges and Schools Commission on Institutions of Higher Education.* Boulder, CO: Naropa Institute, Appendix.

Parry-Jones, W.L. (1981) The model of the Geel Lunatic Colony and its influence on the nineteenth-century asylum system in Britain. In: A. Scull (ed.), *Madhouses, Mad-Doctors, and Madmen.* Philadelphia: University of Pennsylvania Press.

Perceval, J. (1961) *Perceval's Narrative: A Patient's Account of His Psychosis* (ed. Gregory Bateson). Stanford, CA: Stanford University Press.

Podvoll, E. (1980) The psychotic journey. 1: Psychotic states of mind. *Naropa Institute Journal of Psychology*, **1**: 21–31.

Podvoll, E. (1983) Megalomania: psychotic predicament and transformation. *Naropa Institute Journal of Psychology*, **2**: 64–83.

Podvoll, E. (1985) Protecting recovery from psychosis in home environments. *Naropa Institute Journal of Psychology*, **3**: 71–89.

Pollack, P. *et al.* (1977) Treating the insane in sane places. *Journal of Community Psychology*, **5**: 380–387.

Searles, H. (1979a) The 'dedicated physician' in the field of psychotherapy and psychoanalysis. In: *Countertransference and Related Subjects*. New York: International University Press.

Searles, H. (1979b) The patient as therapist to his analyst. In: *Countertransference and Related Subjects*. New York: International University Press.

Trungpa, C. (1978) *Glimpses of Abhidharma*. Boulder, CO: Prajna Press.

Trungpa, C. (1983) Creating an environment of sanity. *Naropa Institute Journal of Psychology*, **2**: 1–10.

Trungpa, C. (1984) *Shambhala: the Sacred Path of the Warrior*. Boston, MA: Shambhala Publications.

Trungpa, C. (1985) Acknowledging death as the common ground of healing. *Naropa Institute Journal of Psychology*, **3**: 3–10.

Introduction to Chapter 14

Shaun Parsons and Alan Armstrong

by Phil Barker

In this chapter Shaun Parsons and Alan Armstrong mount a spirited defence of the 'responsible' use of power and authority in psychiatry. In doing so, they draw as much on their own humanity as they do upon an appreciation of the methodological basis of classification and the philosophical background to the whole orientation to people in psychiatric distress.

Shaun Parsons is a Lecturer in Psychiatric Nursing Practice at the University of Newcastle, where he received his doctorate. He is a registered mental and a registered general nurse, as well as a Chartered Psychologist. One of his long-term research interests has been people with a diagnosis of personality disorder and his doctoral research focused on the validity of the concept of the DSM IV Cluster B Personality Disorders, within Primary Health Care. He draws on some of that background here, as he argues that psychiatric classification is an essential feature of modern psychiatry. His current clinical and research work is concentrated on forensic psychiatry where he is particularly interested in psychiatric morbidity within prison populations and how people with psychiatric disorders are treated within the criminal justice system.

Alan Armstrong is also a registered nurse who presently is a doctoral candidate at the University of Newcastle, under the supervision of Phil Barker and Shaun Parsons. His first degree was in philosophy and he gained his MA in Health Care Ethics from the University of Leeds. Ethical issues are Alan's main interest, and he explores this, in part, within this chapter. His doctoral research is focused on the role of virtue ethics in psychiatric nursing, particularly in relation to decision-making in practice.

This chapter provides a fitting conclusion to Part Two, serving as a provocative 'book end' to Thomas Szasz's opening essay in Part One. Shaun and Alan try not only to defend some of the traditional concepts associated with psychiatric care and treatment, but also try to embed their defence within an appreciation of a world of health care which is very much in flux, and which may need a sense of stability, in order to function. Their main argument focuses on the moral duties owed by psychiatric professionals to their patients and how such functions might, ultimately, be to the greater good of those who need psychiatric services.

14

Psychiatric power and authority: a scientific and moral defence

Shaun Parsons and Alan Armstrong

INTRODUCTION

In this book the concepts of psychiatric power and authority have been examined and called into question. Authors such as Szasz, Boyle and Coleman have contended that power is abused, and furthermore, they argue that the concepts of power and authority are incorrectly located within the realm of psychiatry. This contention is generally made on the basis of two premises. First, that psychiatric diagnoses are socially constructed entities, which have no basis in reality and are flawed in construction. This argument is most eloquently proposed by Boyle in Chapter 5. Secondly, Szasz (Chapter 3) argues that psychiatric services have no legitimacy to exercise power over individuals, and therefore, involuntary psychiatric interventions are morally indefensible. We do not accept these contentions. We will argue that psychiatric diagnoses, whilst not completely reliable, are important, necessary and valuable constructs for both clinical and moral reasons in psychiatric practice. Our argument on this latter point centres on the strict obligations of beneficence and non-maleficence which psychiatrists owe toward their patients.

PSYCHIATRIC CLASSIFICATION AND DIAGNOSIS

Diagnosis and classification are used by psychiatrists and psychologists to make sense of patients' presenting symptoms and complaints. Classification is not unique to psychiatry but is found in all sciences. Indeed all humans use classification in everyday life. For example an animal that has four legs, a wet nose, barks and enjoys walks is classified as a dog. This decision (or classification) has only been arrived at by looking at the attributes and features of the animal and assigning it a category. The purpose of the categorization or classification is to communicate the meaning of a given construct thus avoiding the need to repeat a detailed description of objects when an object is referred to. An essential feature of this premise is that when X says that a dog was seen, Y has a mental image of a hairy creature with a wet nose, four legs and a tail and which also barks. Similarly chemists and physicists classify elements on a periodic table by their molecular weight. These scientists are building a concept or construct of physical objects by describing its properties: coal is hard and black, oxidizes exothermically and is made of carbon. Psychologists and psychiatrists use a similar but not identical way of classifying. The symptoms of mental illness are mediated through the mirror of the subject's personality, experience and viewpoint. Classification in psychiatry is an attempt to impose order and meaning, using (arguably) objective observation, on the diaspora of psychiatric symptomatology. As such the process of classification in psychiatry and psychology is controversial and problematic.

In addition psychiatric classification serves a number of practical functions. In a world where, increasingly, health and social welfare provision is limited by budgetary restraints psychiatric classification is a key element in resource planning and allocation. Epidemiological data on, for example, affective disorders or schizophrenia allows resources to be planned and allocated to mental health services. From the patient's perspective psychiatric classification helps to decide levels of sickness benefits, certified sick time away from work and access to psychiatric and mental health services.

Psychiatric classification: a brief history

The first record of mental disorder can be found in 3000 BC in Egypt when Prince Ptah-hotep was diagnosed as having what would now be recognized as Alzheimer's disease. By 1400 BC descriptions of melancholia and hysteria can be found which would be recognizable as their DSM IV equivalents today (Mack *et al.*, 1994).

Hippocrates in 460–377 BC devised six types of mental disorders:

1 Phrenitis (acute mental disturbance with confusion)
2 Mania (acute mental disturbance without fever)
3 Melancholia (all chronic mental disturbance)
4 Epilepsy (which has survived unchanged)
5 Hysteria (paroxysmic dysponea, pain and convulsions)
6 Scythian disease (transvestism)

Hippocrates also devised four temperaments:

1 Choleric (angry)
2 Sanguine (optimistic, cheerful)
3 Melancholic (pessimistic, depressed)
4 Phlegmatic (apathetic, indifferent)

Hippocrates arrived at these classifications by observing patients and their symptoms and grouping like symptoms together. Hippocrates' system of classification can be called a descriptive system as are both DSM IV and ICD-10.

Plato also developed a classification system based upon logical or rational conceptualizations. Plato split mental disorder into two categories: Illness based upon physical problems and illness given by divine gift. Plato did not define mental illness by the presenting symptoms but by his assumed underlying causes of the disorder. As such, symptoms were a secondary consideration in Plato's system. An equivalent today would be a stroke caused by damage to the brain by haemorrhage or ischaemia. Such a system can be called an aetiological system. The aetiological classification of disease operates through most of physical medicine today.

The evolution of modern classification

Modern psychiatric classification has its origins in eighteenth century France when the popularity of science increased interest in psychiatric classification (Mack *et al.*, 1994). The rise of science included the adoption of a scientific method, which would become known as positivism. The central philosophy of positivistic classification was defined by Goldstein as: 'The classification of data under clear and distinct rubrics' (Goldstein, 1988 cited by Mack *et al.*, 1994). In other words, the objective observation and classification of clusters of symptoms to hypothetical disorders which are then amenable to 'scientific' investigation. Within the positivist enquiry were certain implicit and explicit beliefs: that nature was uniform and consistent; diseases were distinct and separate entities and that it is possible to observe objectively (Sydenham, ([1682]1848). Mack *et al.* (1994) quotes Sydenham as saying that 'the physician should consider observation carefully and that empirical data should be *sorted by patterns of co-occurrence* much as a botanist classifying plants' (emphasis added). Here Sydenham is describing a descriptive classification system based upon the hypothesis that diseases are distinct and produce discrete and classifiable pathology and symptoms. Sydenham was arguing for the same methodology used in the present DSM IV and ICD-10 classification systems and which has come to be described as the Linnaen system after the Swedish botanist who developed a descriptive classification system for the science of botany.

The scientific and positivist trend continued throughout the eighteenth and nineteenth centuries. However, there were conflicts between proponents of Sydenham's descriptive model of classification and proponents of a more Platonic classification based upon aetiology. There were continuing attempts to adopt an aetiological model when Bayle in 1822 attempted to link psychiatric symptoms with brain lesions. The approach yielded some early understanding of the aetiology of strokes and what later became known as Alzheimer's disease, but in general, despite a revival of interest in neuroscience, the descriptive methodology remained dominant. This was mainly because there was little aetiological knowledge available to researchers due to their relatively primitive enquiries, despite frequent autopsies of deceased patients.

In late nineteenth century psychiatry Charcot was one of the most prominent and ardent describer of symptoms and was influential in the consolidation of the descriptive system. Charcot described in considerable detail the symptoms associated with psychiatric disorder and particularly hysteria. Charcot took particular pride in his 'practising nosology': his interest in naming 'the apparent chaos presented by the continual repetition of the same symptoms . . . [which] . . . then gave way to order' (Freud, 1893, cited in Mack *et al.*, 1994).

Kraepelin (1896) used Sydenham's and Charcot's descriptive methods to produce the first modern classification system when he hypothesized that all patients whose symptoms had the same course had the same disease, a view that has remained central to DSM IV and ICD-10. Kraepelin produced a textbook of psychiatry in which he named disorders based upon descriptions of symptoms. The table of contents of Kraepelin's textbook was the foundation of modern psychiatric classification. Kraepelin's view was not universally accepted, with some researchers continuing to argue for an aetiological system. Meyer, for example, argued for an aetiological classification system built upon reactions (Mack *et al.*, 1994), whilst Hill (1907) mocked the US classification system, particularly the number of new disorders, which he saw as absurd. At the same time statistical information and the need for an epidemiology of psychiatric morbidity began to have an effect on classification, particularly in the United States. These pressures have continued to grow over time and are perhaps the most powerful driving force behind classification in psychiatry. A tension began to develop between the need for psychiatric classification for practical purposes against the need for a diagnostically accurate classification system, which continues to the present day.

To address the need for statistical and epidemiological information the American Medico-Psychological Association and the National Committee for Mental Hygiene devised a list of twenty-two psychiatric diseases for use across all institutions in the US. Their classification was developed through the 1920s and 1930s into the Standard Classification. The Standard Classification was superseded by US military classifications that had grown during the Second World War to include the post-traumatic disorders. After the war the American Psychiatric Association (APA) reviewed existing classifications and published DSM I in 1952 (APA, 1952). DSM I, and to a lesser extent ICD-6, elevated the importance of diagnosis which was seen as a cornerstone of the practice of psychiatric medicine (Raines, 1952 cited in Mack *et al.*, 1994). Raines also argued that DSM I should be flexible enough to allow for change of existing disorders and inclusion of new disorders. Raines was in fact arguing for DSM as a heuristic, descriptive and pragmatic system of hypothesized disorders. The APA accepted the importance of Raines's argument and in addition wished to produce a diagnostic system that comprised of descriptions of symptoms which were atheoretical in nature in order to facilitate research and to enhance communication across disciplines with different philosophical bases (Mack *et al.*, 1994). This aim was first realized with the publication of DSM III (APA, 1980). DSM III was produced by committees, which reviewed the previous research for each proposed classification. Based upon the empirical findings, symptoms were assigned to diagnostic categories in the form of descriptive operational criteria. Each of these criteria was amenable to further research and validity and reliability testing. Indeed the trend towards a classification system, which is based upon empirical data, made the revision of DSM III, DSM III-R (APA, 1987) necessary and has led to the latest DSM, DSM IV (APA, 1994).

We can see that from the above brief history the APA has devised a descriptive classification system, which is produced through a review of previous empirical research *and is then, tested and reviewed through ongoing research.* The methodology used to construct the DSMs is therefore positivist and empiricist in nature. However, this methodology has been described as flawed and rejected by Boyle earlier in this book. Boyle is occupying a position which we will describe as nominalist whilst an opposing position can be described as realist. These tensions will now be explored.

Nominalism versus realism

Essentially, the nominalist position states that 'nothing especially psychiatric disorders exists except as it is constructed in the minds of people' (Frances *et al.*, 1994). In other words the idea that psychiatric diagnoses are social constructions devised to serve political, social and professional interests. The extreme nominalist position expressed by Boyle (1990), and earlier in this book, is that 'disorders' are constructs derived by faulty 'scientific' method and are not based upon real phenomena.

The realists' viewpoint is reductionist. Realists argue that the classification, for example, of schizophrenia actually represents a disorder with a biological substrate, much in the same way that the signs and symptoms of chickenpox or measles represents an underlying viral infection. The realist view depends on being able to find an underlying pathology to the symptomatology described in the classification. Each of these positions will be briefly examined.

In her earlier chapter and in her 1990 book *Schizophrenia a Scientific Delusion*, Boyle has contended that mental illness is classified in a different way from physical illness and the natural sciences. Boyle argued that there are clear rules for the construction of scientific constructs. These are 'correspondence rules based on prior observation of patterns and not on the post hoc deliberations of committees' Boyle (1990: 170). Boyle states that the concept of mental illness is abstract and is a construction rather than a representation of a real event or disorder. When Boyle states 'if reliable criteria for inferring a diagnostic label have to be sought, then the label should not have been brought into existence' (see Chapter 5 above, p. 75), she is arguing that in psychiatry the observable phenomena are fitted into constructs which have been previously defined. The subject's symptoms are fitted into the construct rather than the symptoms defining the construct and therefore, Boyle argues, can never be valid or reliable. Boyle describes this process as flawed because she denies the reality of an underlying disorder. A contention she supports by pointing to the lack of aetiological evidence for psychiatric disorders. As she says, 'you can't expect researchers, however well funded, to identify the processes which hold together a non-existent pattern' (p. 75). A similar point was made by Malmgren (1993) who argues that DSM III and DSM IV are based upon out dated theories of positivist empiricist meaning based upon operational definition of symptom criteria. If accepted, Malmgren's argument means that DSM IV is flawed at a fundamental level because of a need to classify operational criteria in a descriptive way.

The nominalist position, including Boyle, has been criticized. For example, Monach (1995), reviewing Boyle's work on schizophrenia, raises the point that the development of theory and constructs in many natural sciences would also not meet Boyle's rigid nosological criteria. A number of natural sciences have used observable and subjective phenomena to derive theory. Carl Linnaeus (1707–78), in many ways the father of positivistic classification, used precisely this method in his book *Sytema naturae Fundamenta Botanica, Genera Plantarum, Critica Botanica*. With this book Linnaeus founded botanical classification using a descriptive, observationally based classification. Similar classifications were adopted by zoology and biology and in these sciences the descriptive approach has led to errors, for example sharks and dolphins were thought to be related because they looked alike. However, the approach has also led to many practical and useful theories and methodologies. Perhaps the best example is Newton's theory of gravity. Newton used mathematical constructs to provide a mathematical description of the effects of gravity that could be observed in the universe. Newton provided a theory of gravitation with many practical day-to-day uses. Yet Newton's underlying theory of the nature of gravity and space-time was flawed as Einstein, Hawking and others have since shown. Despite this fundamental flaw, Newtonian gravitational mathematics is still taught and used to explain everyday motion and gravitational effects to this day; the mathematical constructs are so descriptively useful they have survived the destruction of their underlying theory. In terms of psychiatric classification the usefulness of the description in identifying caseness, meaning whether a disorder is present or not, and predicating treatment course may be the most useful feature of the classification. It is, perhaps, a fault with Boyle's argument and nominalism generally that this practical Linnean tradition in classification is not accepted.

The realist position is most often expressed by neuroscience and biological psychiatry (for example Gorwood *et al.*, 1996). It is a realist reductionist philosophy that drives the search for a 'schizophrenia' gene or biological markers for depression. To an extreme realist the disorders in DSM are not heuristic concepts but confirmed disease entities. The DSM III-R and DSM IV task forces did not intend the DSMs to be used this way. Frances, a member of the DSM IV task force, describes the realist view as naive arguing that DSM IV was intended to be heuristic and pragmatic and that the disorders and criteria were intended to be hypotheses which could be used for clinical work and as a framework for further research towards an aetiological classification system (Frances *et al.*, 1994). Frances argues that realists must acknowledge this fact.

A further criticism of realism has been made by Kendler (1990), who argues that realists rely on the empiricist scientific method which can only answer 'little' questions. In a paper defending DSM IV, Frances points out that this is a narrow view of science and empiricism (Frances *et al.*, 1994). Frances argues that science has always been more than pure empiricism; citing Lakatos (1978), Frances argues that science involves empiricism (hypothesis testing) and rationalism (the formulation of theories and formation of hypotheses). Frances goes on to say that 'interpretation, discussion, disagreement and debate concerning the ambiguity and relevance of empirical finding is integral to the scientific method'. Frances is arguing that empiricism is more than just experimentation it also involves setting the results in a wider framework and applying them to the social world. Frances is arguing that the nosological process, which Boyle condemns, is a strength rather than a weakness of classification.

The above points also highlight the point of the value of descriptive and aetiological systems. Mack *et al.* (1994) state that even Kraepelin hoped that one day there would be an aetiologically based system. In theory such a system would not have to deal with heuristic concepts but with biologically based certainties. A review of the literature also makes clear that modern psychiatric knowledge is not yet in this position. There remains wide disagreement over biological markers for, for example, Affective disorders, Schizophrenia and Personality Disorder (Akiskal, 1994; Kirov and Murray, 1997). Mack *et al.* quote Earle, a nineteenth century psychiatrist, who wrote 'In the present state of our knowledge, no classification of insanity can be erected upon a pathological basis, for the simple reason that, with few exceptions, the pathology of the disease is unknown . . . we are forced to fall back upon the symptomatology of the disease' (Earle, quoted by Mack *et al.*, 1994: 520). The situation although improved *and improving* has, for many psychiatric disorders, not changed today and Mack *et al.* (1994) go on to agree with Frances *et al.* (1994) that the DSMs are intended as way-stations to an aetiological classification system – which at present is a hope rather than a reality.

To conclude: a review of the literature leads us to the conclusion that at present there is no resolution to the debate between nominalism and realism for two main reasons:

1 There is a lack of biological markers to the constructs of mental disorders in psychiatric classification. This is due to either inadequate knowledge of the brain and the pathology underlying the disorders *and/or* the fact that the constructs are false and no such markers exist.
2 Due in part to the first reason, psychiatric classifications remain heuristic constructs.

Point 1 undermines the realist position since repeated searches for biological markers have produced negative or ambiguous results; for example the inconclusive biological evidence for depression and personality disorder (Gold and Silk, 1993) or the still controversial evidence for genetic markers for schizophrenia (Gorwood *et al.*, 1997). However, the two papers quoted above also undermine the nominalist view since both reviews point to a large amount of biological evidence which, whilst inconclusive, could be construed as suggestive of some kind of common biological substrate in each disorder. In addition, these papers are only two examples drawn from a vast literature of similar papers.

It is the last point that Boyle fails to adequately dismiss in her arguments. Boyle dismisses all of psychiatric diagnosis as not meeting her strict nosological standards but fails to adequately explain why psychiatric diagnoses should have common features or any predictive reliability or validity. Yet, for example, Gorwood *et al.* (1997) find some evidence for biological foundations for schizophrenia. This example and others like it cannot be simply explained away as coincidences. If there is no underlying construct then any kind of consistent commonality should be absent: it is not.

In addition, we see the biggest failure of the nomanalists, including Boyle, as being the failure to adequately explain how abandoning current psychiatric diagnoses, or the empiricist positivist process upon which they are based, would improve matters. Other critics agree: for example, Monach (1995) states, when reviewing Boyle's (1990) work *Schizophrenia: a Scientific Delusion,* that 'there is little to suggest from her analysis [of schizophrenia] that abandoning the term schizophrenia will in itself achieve more humane and appropriate mental health services' (Monach, 1995: 194). People expect to be given a diagnosis and the mechanisms through which they obtain benefits and arrange time away from work all demand a diagnosis. It is hard to see how these essential systems could operate within another paradigm. Diagnosis therefore fulfils a useful and essential role in our society, one we argue that must be acknowledged by nominalists.

A compromise

Where does this leave the researcher or clinician who wishes to use psychiatric classification in clinical practice or research? We would agree with the APA in arguing for a middle way. The APA admits that these issues remain unresolved (Frances *et al.*, 1994), but argue that DSM IV is a heuristic and pragmatic classification system. Frances clarifies this position, arguing that the DSMs are an attempt to form a middle ground between realism and nominalism and that 'mental disorders are better conceived as no more than *(but also no less than)* valuable heuristic constructs' (Frances *et al.*, 1994: 210). Frances argues (and we agree) that it is important not to underestimate the clinical and research value of heuristic diagnostic concepts or the value of these constructs in predicting course, family history, treatment response and future health trends/ demands. In short, we are arguing for a pragmatic approach where DSM IV constructs are accepted as heuristic criteria, and are treated as such. From the position of pragmatism, it is legitimate, indeed essential, to research the structure, diagnostic criteria, epidemiology and aetiology of each disorder as long as the results are used to continually test the validity and usefulness of the diagnosis. If the diagnosis is found wanting it could be changed, adapted or discarded and replaced with a new or refined hypothesis which explains the phenomenon more completely than its predecessor. In short, a positivist empiricist approach of hypothesis testing.

We accept the approach and underlying philosophy of DSM IV because of its pragmatic usefulness, amenability to research and acceptance of the fundamental human need to classify. It is this final point that is felt to be most important, as classification is a common part of every day life. There are essential human, societal and political needs to name objects and events in our lives, needs that nominalists ignore.

We believe that often a diagnosis can be the starting point for useful and effective intervention and research and can be a therapeutic and useful starting point in a treatment plan from both the patient's and clinician's point of view.

In the next section four moral arguments to support involuntary psychiatric interventions will be examined. We discuss Szasz's argument against these types of practices and critique this where appropriate.

ARGUMENTS SUPPORTING INVOLUNTARY PSYCHIATRIC INTERVENTIONS

There are several moral arguments that could be employed in order to support the justification of involuntary psychiatric interventions. For the purposes of this chapter, these are: the argument from liberty; the rights-based argument; the duty-based argument; and the personal identity/interests based argument. These will now be examined.

The argument from liberty

According to Hospers (1974: p. 212), libertarianism

> [is] the doctrine that every person is the owner of his own life, and that no one is the owner of anyone else's life: and that consequently every human being has the right to act in accordance with his own choices, unless those infringe on the equal liberty of other human beings to act in accordance with their choices.

A classic work of this ideology can be found in J. S. Mill's *On Liberty*. Here Mill refutes the legitimacy of the state to intervene in the personal lives of individuals. However, he defends the view that the state has a moral obligation to protect its citizens from the potential danger, injury and harm that might result from someone deemed to be dangerous to others. Many psychiatrists agree with this moral position. 'Insiders' (as Szasz refers to them) may defend involuntary detention, suggesting that it is just and fair for two reasons: first, the prevention of harm to the innocent and second, the benefits brought to the patient. We argue that the argument from liberty is more appropriately seen as the right to self-determination (more of this in the next section); as such, the majority of people will probably agree with the concept of owning one's own life and making one's own choices. However, the important point is whether or not this still applies when one is deemed, correctly or not, as irrational or 'a danger to oneself or others'.

The rights-based argument

We agree with Szasz when he contends that the language of rights is in vogue. It often appears as though this rhetoric is exaggerated, that 'new' rights are put forward to facilitate and promote those things which we want to enjoy or protect and, in the end, this notion loses some of its legitimacy and force. (Remember, *valid* conclusions to moral problems cannot be reached, as these are the province of deductive reasoning, and moral argument is concerned with inductive reasoning, that is, the conclusion can only be *probably* true.)

It is because of the above that we need to be clear about the authority and origin of each moral right used to resolve moral dilemmas. Do we think that all individuals in every circumstance have a right to treatment; and conversely a right to refuse treatment? If we think the latter, is this because we always accept that an individual has a right to self-determination? What is the relationship between rationality and making autonomous decisions? What degree of reasoning/rationality (a difficult concept to define usefully) is required to be present for someone to refuse, what appears to be, a sensible, necessary and, perhaps even, a life-saving treatment? Questions like these need to be addressed in a responsible way, involving a multi-disciplinary approach. We need to ensure that an individual who chooses (or refuses) a treatment/therapy etc. (where others regard this as unconventional) is not necessarily labelled and categorized as irrational. Humans have unique value systems, not to mention cultural differences; both these factors, and more, are involved in moral decision-making. We believe that unless mental illness is diagnosed, individuals have a right (however, is this absolute, strict or merely weak and prima facie?) to refuse even life-saving treatments. Examples of this kind include terminally ill patients who refuse yet another chemotherapy regime. However, it is difficult to weigh the right to self-determination against the sanctity of human life, undoubtedly a socially pragmatic concept. For example, how many individuals who having been prevented from committing suicide, are now living better, more useful and happier lives? Care needs to be taken concerning these types of decisions. For an individual to make an informed choice, he needs to have the capacities of understanding, evaluation and reasoning. This process may sound simple, but in practice, it requires expert medical and nursing care, especially effective communication (particularly listening skills) between psychiatrists and patients.

Szasz's antipathy toward 'force' and 'psychiatric power' implies an assumption, on his part, that these are necessarily and intrinsically bad things. Does he believe this because human rights are not respected? If so, there is scant evidence of this belief, and no structured argument to support this. If it is the case that Szasz frowns upon disrespecting rights, then is he just inconsistent in his attitude toward an individual's right to treatment when ill?

Regarding the pragmatism of moral rights, let us first look at Szasz's argument. This can be presented thus:

Premise 1 (P1):   'mental illness' does not exist.

Premise 2 (P2):   the concept of mental illness is a social and evaluative construct.

Conclusion: therefore, psychiatric services have no legitimacy to exercise power, for example, the involuntary detention of individuals.

For the sake of argument, let us accept his thesis about mental illness. Surely the point is that these people *are* distressed; their well-being is affected in a detrimental way, and their lives are less happy than perhaps they could be. Whether these phenomena are caused by society, are socially constructed concepts or have a biochemical origin, would Szasz deny these people the right to treatments that, in many cases, would lessen their distress by relieving symptoms and thus improving overall well-being?

At one point, Szasz acknowledges the 'pain and suffering' (see p. 46) that individuals are vulnerable to. It is, in part, in order to minimize or prevent these negative emotions that we think that moral decision-making in psychiatry ought to be guided by one or more moral concepts. Besides moral rights, these can include the following: 'principles' such as, the principle of beneficence, moral duties, consequences of acts/ omissions and the cultivation of moral virtues (the latter two are not discussed here). This is important since psychiatry is an evaluative and descriptive practice. It is not an exact science (although neither is physical medicine, but at least this is more aetiologically based). Experts classify psychiatric disorders from symptoms and histories. Besides diagnosing mental disease, there are problems with the notion of mental competence. Whilst in essence a legal concept, it is interrelated with the notion of an individual's decision-making capacity. Both of these are graded concepts, certainly not black and white and difficult for psychiatrists to agree upon. These human processes are moral; each step involves making decisions, choosing between options, weighing up the pros and cons of alternatives and ultimately, attempting to do what is right and good for each individual.

Regarding the principle of respecting the autonomous decisions of individuals, Szasz fails to develop any specific moral argument based upon this. He does not even mention 'medical paternalism', which, according to Matthews, is 'The sense of the imposition of treatment upon a patient against the patient's will, because the *doctor* regards it as in the patient's best interests' (1994: p. 103).

The 'even' was intentional; paternalism is the notion most referred to in psychiatric ethics when there are conflicts between obligations of beneficence and respect for autonomy. Why does Szasz neglect this important notion? If one rejects his initial premise (P1) then his conclusion is not inevitable. He perhaps should at least take this notion (paternalism) into account; likewise, other moral concepts, such as, 'autonomy' and 'respect for autonomy' only receive scant attention.

The duty-based argument

For those, such as the authors, who do not *fully* accept the usefulness of invoking the notion of moral rights, what alternative moral concepts are there which can be more pragmatically invoked? One response to this question is to turn to the notion of moral duties. The hope being that a clearer picture emerges regarding the reasoning behind justifiable involuntary interventions. Why might this be? Firstly, there are professional codes of conduct governing the medical and psychiatric professions. These essentially aim to provide guidelines for good (research and evidence-based) clinical and ethical practice. Besides legal duties which the psychiatrist owes to his patients (and which are punishable in law if not performed), there are certain moral duties which he owes to each patient under his care. For some, these duties can simply be encompassed under the umbrella slogan 'duty of care'. For others, like the authors, there is a need to clarify this concept. Greater precision is needed as to the exact content, origin and nature of each specific duty. In the same way that there can be strict and weak rights, so there can also be strict and weak duties. We argue that there is a strict duty to treat mentally ill patients who are vulnerable and require medical help. In contemporary medical ethics, the obligations of beneficence (to do good and promote well-being) and non-maleficence (to minimize harms) are of fundamental concern. The latter is regarded as a stricter duty; it is much more important, in morality, to refrain from harming someone than it is to do that person some good. The fact that some duties are considered stricter than others, ought to assist us when there are conflicts between obligations. Ross (1930) discussed the concept of prima facie duties; these are duties 'at first sight'. In any given situation, we are obligated to follow duty X until a stricter duty, Y, comes along. For example, it might be supposed that we have a duty to keep promises. One day we have promised to meet a friend at the cinema. However, on our way, we come across a serious accident and try to help save someone's life. We had a prima facie duty to keep the promise with our friend, but this duty was discharged when we witnessed and stopped at the accident.

Two examples of moral duties are: (A) the duty of a psychiatrist to protect the patient from himself, and (B) the duty of the psychiatrist to protect the public. Both of these figure heavily in one form or another in the current Mental Health Act (1983). Moral duties can be negative or positive; the former means, in general, 'not to do act X'; the latter conversely means that 'act X ought to be carried out'. So in the case of the moral virtue of honesty, a positive duty would imply that no lies were told; whereas, a negative duty would insist that the truth be told. Another example of a strict duty is the duty to refrain from killing; an example of a weaker duty would be the duty to come to a stranger's rescue. It would, in most circumstances, be deemed morally worse for one moral agent to kill another, compared to walking along a riverside and refusing to attempt the rescue of someone seen drowning. In the first example, one would be morally (and legally) responsible and blameworthy, and thus be punishable under criminal law for homicide. Whereas, in the second, although in the eyes of other moral agents one perhaps could be held morally blameworthy, it is not morally obligatory to rescue someone else. Indeed this type of act may even be viewed as being supererogatory: above and beyond what is morally expected from someone in 'normal' circumstances. Returning to examples (A) and (B) above, which one is stricter and why? Depending upon the psychiatrist's personal and moral position concerning, for example, the ethics of suicide and the value of life, the duty to protect patient A from harming himself can be seen to be less obligatory than the duty for the psychiatrist to protect members of the public. This could be explained simply in terms of respecting the self-determination of patient A. As mentioned earlier, each human being (even when thought unwise) has a moral right to refuse treatment; and psychiatrists have corresponding duties to take these into account and respect them. But it is also one of the duties of a psychiatrist to promote the overall well-being of their patients. There will be occasions when rights and duties conflict, and the resolution of these dilemmas depends on several factors, not least, the individual moral 'persuasion' of the psychiatrist. In concluding this section, members of the public are 'innocent' in so far as they have no prior knowledge about patient A. Because of this they fail to understand that patient A is dangerous. No matter how difficult decisions like these are to make, a psychiatrist with this knowledge and the means to be able to act upon this – thus preventing possible injury – has a strict and positive moral duty to involuntarily detain this patient.

The personal identity and interests argument

We have seen that strict moral obligations include the principle of beneficence and the stricter duty of non-maleficence. A common notion, especially in medicine, is 'best interests', which is concerned with promoting what are considered to be the most important physical, psychological and spiritual interests of the patient. In psychiatry, an interesting philosophical notion arises when the mental illness affects personal identity. For example, is the person receiving treatment the same as the person prior to the advent of the illness? If not (perhaps one believes that their values and interests have altered somewhat), whose wishes and desires should one follow and respect? The person at the time of treatment or the person prior to the start of the mental illness? This point is related to the important notion of 'insight', one that is frequently cited in psychiatry, but one that Szasz in his conference paper (Chapter 3) fails to mention once.

The task of identifying a patient's interests and values is not simple; it demands time, attention to detail and considerable clinical and psychosocial expertise. However, psychiatrists ought to be trusted, unless there are good reasons not to, to carry out this process. After all, if someone wants expert legal advice, he will consult a lawyer; when someone wants to buy a house, he will visit an estate agent; and when someone wishes to buy an oil painting, he will visit an art dealer for expert advice. Even more important, therefore, that when a person's mental/physical health is at stake, one is able to receive expert psychiatric/medical consultation. Ordinarily, we would listen to this advice and, in all probability, act according to the doctor's recommendations. However, when someone is suffering from a mental illness, there is a chance that perhaps because of the nature of the disease, he is unable to think rationally and comprehend the implications surrounding treatment. In these situations, we argue, that the psychiatrist's duty is to treat the patient, and if necessary, involuntarily. The aim being to alleviate the symptoms (thought responsible for affecting rationality) as quickly as possible. During this period in hospital, the patient's well-being will be safeguarded and promoted.

It must be stressed that just because a patient is involuntarily detained, this does not mean that all manner of treatments can be forced upon him. There remains the need that the benefits/goods of each treatment, medication and therapy etc. outweigh any likely harms/injury. We disagree with the language ('incarcerate', see p. 51) used by Szasz. If the period of involuntary detention is kept to a minimum (however, as mentioned above, it is important to diagnose, treat, relieve symptoms and rehabilitate), and in the post-detention period the individual behaves, thinks, acts etc. in a more logical, rational and healthier manner, then according to our claims concerning a person's interests, not only will the motive behind the involuntary detention have been morally justified, so too will the actual care.

It is undeniable that psychiatrists, through mental health legislation, have wide-ranging powers. Ideally the hope is for these powers to be exercised appropriately with due care and attention. Unfortunately, there have been occasions, as Szasz points out, when 'psychiatric treatment' has been misused. Innocent individuals, who perhaps are merely 'guilty' of opposing the governing political ideology, have found themselves imprisoned or involuntarily admitted into mental hospitals. Clearly then these acts are morally indefensible, irrespective of which moral theory one invokes.

Szasz argued that the concept of mental illness is a myth (Szasz, 1960). As we have seen (P1 and P2), according to him it was literally devoid of substantive meaning, psychiatric diagnoses lacked any objectivity, and therefore, examples of the abuse of psychiatric power – such as involuntary detention/administration of psychotrophic medications – are to be undermined and judged as morally indefensible.

Szasz's argument against the existence of mental illness with its implications for the morality of involuntary psychiatric interventions, needs to be borne in mind when reviewing his present chapter (Chapter 3). Szasz aims to clarify why he has reached this conclusion about the ethics of involuntary psychiatric interventions. He writes:

> I oppose involuntary psychiatric interventions, not because I believe that they are necessarily 'bad' for patients, but because I oppose using the power of the state to impose psychiatric relations on persons against their will. By the same token, I support voluntary psychiatric interventions, not because I believe that they are necessarily 'good' for patients, but because I oppose the power of the state to interfere with contractual relations between consenting adults (see p. 45 above).

How does Szasz intend to deal with those that others might diagnose as mentally ill? His response is straightforward: 'If the person called "patient" breaks no law, he has a right to liberty. And if he breaks the law, he ought to be adjudicated and punished in the criminal justice system' (see p. 52).

Presumably those who accept P1 and P2 like Szasz, will draw the same, or very similar, conclusions as he does about the ethics of involuntary psychiatric interventions and, therefore, the abuse of psychiatric power. Szasz's use of language is interesting. For instance, the phrase 'the myriad uses of psychiatric coercions' is probably to be expected from someone who holds these premises. However, in general, Szasz fails to defend his thesis. Specifically, he does not adequately explain and justify P1 and P2, and he disregards and ignores possible counter-arguments supporting and justifying involuntary detention, for example.

Are we to think, like Szasz, that it is *always* morally wrong to involuntarily detain someone? Can there never be occasions when it would be the morally right and good thing to do? Is adopting Szasz's conclusion a morally responsible position to take? Like all medico-moral dilemmas, when there is conflict between two or more moral obligations, the decision to commit an individual against his will, to remove his liberty, is naturally difficult to make. These decisions ought not to be simple for any psychiatrist to make; scepticism and concern should arise if this were the case on a regular basis. But where a psychiatrist has arrived at a 'reliable' diagnosis, carried out a complete risk assessment (in order to predict the 'dangerousness' of the patient) and concluded that the patient ought to be involuntarily detained, then his actions are morally (and clinically) justifiable. As we have contended, psychiatrists have strict moral duties to prevent/minimize distress and promote the well-being of their patients. It is necessary to aim to minimize the inevitable misuse of power. This, in part, might be achieved through stringent self and external regulation of psychiatric services. Besides ethical guidelines, extensive, up to date clinical policies, which aim to promote 'best practice' and are evidence-based, ought to be planned, organized and implemented.

Szasz certainly takes issue with the justifactory nature of the state. But where would the legitimation of psychiatric power originate from, if not the state? It is unclear what Szasz thinks about this question. For instance, would he support some specific powers? Or does he wish to see the abolition of mental health legislation *per se*? Imagine the scenario: each psychiatrist could use their own practical reasoning without any supervision, guidance or regulation from the state. On the one hand, there would be no 'state power' (which Szasz appears to object to in principle); on the other hand, all manner of worse abuses of 'personal power' might occur. It is possible to think that state power is intrinsically (for its own sake) good. Whereas, perhaps the majority of people might hold that state power is only instrumentally good. In other words, the good derives from the ends that it is used towards. For example, some may seize power in order to do good, and overturn bad, evil rulers. If acts are carried out with the intention and motive to do good, then the idea of power is not necessarily bad. It can be seen as a means to a particular end. The question then becomes 'if the means to an end is thought of as evil, does that mean that the end – no matter how good, and to how many – ought not be allowed? Referring to the passage from Orwell's *Nineteen Eighty-Four* that Szasz quotes (see p. 53), perhaps the anatomy of power may be better explained as: the aim/ purpose of persecution is to persecute the aim and purpose of torture is to torture; however, the aim and purpose of power could be to do *good*.

Would it not be more constructive to ask how the 'power' of the psychiatrist could be defended and understood in less negative terms? Psychiatrists require legal powers which are sanctioned from their respective governments in order to be able to carry out involuntary interventions. It is morally indefensible when these powers are misused or abused. This reasoning makes sense whether or not one accepts the existence of mental illness. However, for those who defend the concept of mental illness, the salient point is not to assume moral wrongdoing when one is involved in some way in coercing a patient. Rather, the intended aim is to promote the overall well-being of the patient. What are the predicted benefits and goods that treatment might bring to the patient? To his spouse? His relatives? Or the larger community/society? It might be crucial to the physical and psychological interests of the patient, that he is influenced by persuasion. As far as possible psychiatric treatments should be evidence-based and performed by clinically responsible practitioners. This claim about the justification of involuntary interventions may be made, and supported, by both consequentialists and non-consequentialists. Non-consequentialists, perhaps those persuaded by duty/rights-based moral theories, hold that morality is concerned with more than just the goodness or badness of consequences/outcomes which result from human acts, choices and decisions.

CONCLUSION

In conclusion we reject the contention made by Boyle that psychiatric diagnosis is flawed. On the contrary, we believe that the process which produces psychiatric diagnosis is a rigorous and valid method of scientific enquiry into psychiatric distress. Indeed, it is precisely this method which has led to many significant advances in both the natural sciences and psychiatry.

As we reject the argument that psychiatric diagnoses are flawed social constructions, we also cannot accept the argument made by Szasz. The use of psychiatric power and authority needs to be regulated both by external means and by the psychiatrists themselves. If psychiatric diagnoses are made, as we suggest, then we feel that the power and authority that proceeds from this would be of benefit to the majority of those who use psychiatric services, and also, to society in general. However, caution is required to minimize harm and distress to patients, nor should patients be exploited for individual gain or self-interest. We accept the rhetoric and limited pragmatic usefulness of invoking moral rights and the argument from liberty. But nevertheless we wish to promote the force of invoking professional and moral duties when faced with moral dilemmas in psychiatry.

REFERENCES

Akiskal, H.S. (1994) The temperamental borders of affective disorders. *Acta Psychiatrica Scandinavica*, 89 (suppl 379): 32–37.

American Psychiatric Association (1952) *Diagnostic and Statistical Manual of Mental Disorders*. Washington, DC: APA.

American Psychiatric Association (1980) *Diagnostic and Statistical Manual of Mental Disorders*, 3rd edn. Washington, DC: APA.

American Psychiatric Association (1987) *Diagnostic and Statistical Manual of Mental Disorders – Revised*, 3rd edn. rev. Washington, DC: APA.

American Psychiatric Association (1994) *Diagnostic and Statistical Manual of Mental Disorders*, 4th edn. Washington, DC: APA.

Boyle, M. (1990) *Schizophrenia a Scientific Delusion*. London: Routledge.

Frances, A., Mack, A.H., First, M.B., Widiger, T.A., Ross, R., Forman, L. *et al.* (1994) A forum for bioethics and philosophy of medicine. DSM-IV meets philosophy. Foundations of the new nosology. *Journal of Medicine and Philosophy*, 19(3): 204–297.

Gold, L.J. and Silk, K.R. (1993) Exploring The Borderline Personality Disorder-Major Affective Disorder Interface. In: J. Paris (ed.), *Borderline Personality Disorder, etiology and treatment*. Washington, DC: American Psychiatric Association, pp. 39–66.

Gorwood, P., Leboyer, M., Falissard, B., Jay, M., Rouillon, F. and Feingold, J. (1996) Anticipation in schizophrenia: new light on a controversial problem. *American Journal of Psychiatry*, 153(9): 1173–1177.

Hill, A. (1907) Presidential Address. *American Journal of Insanity*, 64: 1–8.

Hospers, J. ([1974]1998) Libertarianism. In: James P. Sterba (ed.), *Ethics: the Big Questions*. Oxford: Blackwell, pp. 212–222.

Kendler, K. (1990) Towards a scientific psychiatric nosology: strengths and limitations. *Archives of General Psychiatry*, **47**: 969–73.

Kirov, G. and Murray, R. (1997) The molecular genetics of schizophrenia: progress so far. *Molecular Medicine Today*, 3(3): 124–130.

Kraepelin, E. (1896) *Psychiatrie*, 6th edn. Leipzig: Ambr. Abel.

Mack, A.H., Forman, L., Brown, R. and Frances, A. (1994) A brief history of psychiatric classification. *Psychiatric Clinics of North America*, 17(3): 515–523.

Malmgren, H. (1993) Psychiatric classification and empiricist theories of meaning. *Acta Psychiatrica Scandinavica*, 88 (suppl 373): 48–64.

Matthews, E. (1994) Paternalism, care and mental illness. In: A. Grubb (ed.), *Decision-Making and Problems of Incompetence*. Chichester: Wiley & Son, pp. 103–114.

Mill, J.S. (1859) *On Liberty*. London: J.W. Parker & Son.

Monach, J. (1995) Schizophrenia: a scientific delusion (Book Review). *Journal of Psychiatric and Mental Health Nursing*, 2: 191–198.

Ross, W.D. (1930) *The Right and the Good*. Oxford: Clarendon Press.

Sydenham, T. ([1642]1848) Observations Medicae (Preface to edn 3). In: R.G. Latham (trans.), *The Works of Thomas Sydenham*, vol. 3. London: The Sydenham Society.

Szasz, T. (1960) The myth of mental illness. *American Psychologist*, 15: 113–118.

Conclusion

15

History, truth and the politics of madness

Phil Barker

THE END IS THE BEGINNING OF A RELATIONSHIP

Much of this text has focused on psychiatrists. This appears appropriate, not only because much of the power and authority associated with psychiatry is linked to psychiatrists *per se*, but also because this group is the core psychiatric discipline, in influence if not in numbers. Other disciplines describe themselves as psychiatric nurses, psychiatric social workers, or psychiatric aides. Psychiatrists do not call themselves psychiatric physicians. The psychiatrist is the professional enactment of psychiatry.

It is also noteworthy that, as other disciplines rush to redefine themselves as mental health nurses, or workers, psychiatrists show no similar move to redefine their territory. This may be appropriate since, despite the various critiques included in this text, the historian from one hundred years hence might look back on twentieth century psychiatry more favourably than we do at present. This period may have witnessed all manner of pomposity and professional self-deception. It may also have provided a more secure basis for the development of new stages in the human project: extending some of our age-old wisdom into new and potentially more profitable waters.

The psychiatrist is emblematic of all the professions who are threaded through the tapestry of psychiatric history. The psychiatrist engages with people in mental distress and also signifies much of the relationship upon which such engagement is predicated. Thomas (1997) has written of his engagement with a woman, Sharon Lefevre, who cut her arms very badly. On first encountering her he recalled that: 'My heart sank, because I had little experience of helping people who self-harmed, and I really did not know what I was going to do to help her (1997: 232). Thomas began to see her as an out-patient, where they mostly talked about her problems, and his response to them as a doctor. Some months later LeFevre offered to write a play about their relationship, inviting Thomas to perform it with her at a conference in Holland. The play featured a woman in an in-patient ward whose monologue about the state of the world is interrupted by the arrival of a stranger, who turns out to be a psychiatrist. The play subsequently pursues the relationship between the two, in particular the psychiatrist's exasperation with her self-harming, something he has never been able to understand. Ultimately, the psychiatrist begins to move beyond his professional boundary, talking of his own unsatisfactory relationship with his father. However, as he gets close to revealing something important about himself, his professional barriers go up again. The patient notices and comments on this barrier, and the play ends with both discussing whether they can ever really trust one another.

Reflecting on his experience as the actor in the play, Thomas viewed the psychiatrist's barriers as a:

> consequence of the medical drive to control, to exercise knowledge and power. Psychiatrists often talk about boundaries in their relationships with their patients. Boundaries and barriers are closely related. Whether you regard a boundary as a barrier depends on who is in control, and on which side you are situated. (1997: 234)

This observation is critical, since much of psychiatric theory and practice has been predicated on the subject–object relationship. The psychiatrist (representative of all the disciplines) views the patient as an object, exploring his subjective experience of the object, in an effort to draw some meaningful conclusions about 'what is going on' within the person-object. Although most psychiatric professionals try to put themselves in the patient's shoes, empathy rarely moves beyond a special kind of voyeurism. 'The psychiatrist (and all his colleagues) cannot escape the need to observe' (Thomas, 1997: 235).

Cawley (1993) has argued that there are six axioms, or self-evident truths, which are independent of science, and central to human relationships. Cawley's axioms appear to involve a re-working of many of the principles upon which Sullivan based his theory of interpersonal relations (Evans, 1996). For example:

- each person has direct experience of his/her unique self (self-awareness);
- subjective experiences (intrapersonal processes) are of central importance as aspects of the unique self;
- transactions between people (interpersonal processes) constitute a major set of life experiences, as do interactions with other environmental influences (adapted from Cawley, 1993).

Ironically, although in Cawley's view the relationship between the psychiatrist and patient lies 'at the heart of psychiatry', many patients' experiences suggest that such relationships are either fleeting, or grossly unsatisfying (Rogers *et al.*, 1993). Increasingly, similar criticisms are made of nurses, who spend more time on paperwork than they do with patients (Barker, 1999). Despite such reservations, Thomas's – and Cawley's – attempt to extend our appreciation of the need to review the boundaries of psychiatry emphasizes the extent to which the 'truth' of the patient's experience is, at least in part, a function of the psychiatric professional's engagement with that experience. The use of Jasperian phenomenology involves the patient being viewed by a detached observer. This needs to be replaced by a phenomenology of intersubjectivity. Psychiatric professionals might care to begin to consider the extent to which their view of the patient – complete with all its attached status, power and authority – influences the 'object' which is viewed. This point is passé in quantum physics where the plight of Schrödinger's cat, suspended between life and death until the observer observes it, is taken for granted (Zohar, 1991). To what extent are psychiatric professionals aware that the phenomenon – which is the 'the patient' – is, at least in part, a function of their engagement with the patient. When he encountered Sharon LeFevre, Thomas found – to his emotional cost – that his identity as a psychiatrist was as much a function of what she (Sharon) brought to the relationship, as what he had brought of his personal and professional 'selves'. His appreciation of this intersubjective perspective on the professional–user relationship was, however, only a step beyond Sullivan's (1953) dictum: ' everyone is much more simply human than otherwise'. It is worth recalling that Sullivan made this (self-revelatory) observation within the context of his work with people in psychosis in the days long before the introduction of the phenothiazines. The intersubjective perspective implies, however, 'the death of certainty', for one characteristic of relationships is their tidal nature. Psychiatric professionals may discover that they are involved in a process of change, as much as are the people in their care; although it would be folly to forget who is meant to be the 'patient' and who the 'helper'. We should not forget, either, the dangers associated with the adoption of a relationship, which acknowledges the mutuality of human experience. One view of the relative obscurity of Sullivan's work, and the relative demise of one of his direct descendants, RD Laing, has been attributed to the threat to orthodoxy – and the certainty principle – which their mutual relationship with patients necessitated (Kotowicz, 1996).

THE FULFILMENT OF DIRE PREDICTIONS

Although views on the professional–user, interpersonal relationship are, at least, as old as Sullivan, many of the critiques and alternatives perspectives offered in this text, have involved a consideration of patients from a safe (emotional and experiential) distance. Traditionally, the compassion for the 'patients' is derived from the humanitarian ethic. Certainly, it has long been assumed that – at least in Christian terms – we all are our 'brother's keeper' and have a responsibility to care for – and safeguard – those with mental illness.

In a paper first published in 1986, Kathleen Jones, Professor of Social Policy, at the University of York, England, commented on her first-hand observations of the changes to Italian psychiatry, generated by Psichiatria Democratica. That movement had based itself on three main principles – the re-introduction of people with mental illness back into the mainstream of the community; the end to their occupational exploitation; and 'anti-professionalism' – an emphasis on human relations and simple group skills, over professional forms of training. It should not be forgotten that this psychiatric philosophy owed much to the Marxist critique, popular in Italian communism of the period.

Jones was one of the strongest critics of the Italian reformation of its psychiatric system, to emerge in the mid-1980s. She believed that Franco Basaglia, and his followers, had mistaken the response to a problem for its cause:

> mental illness, unfortunately, is not created by mental hospitals (though bad mental hospitals can exacerbate it by outdated institutional practices). Nor is it abolished by simply pretending that it does not exist. Just as water finds its own level, social distress which is denied one outlet will find others. (Jones, 1998: 226)

Jones went on to make a dire prediction of the likely effect of the deinstitutionalization process, should mental hospitals be 'substantially reduced or abolished'. In Jones's view the following was likely to occur:

- The number of single homeless people with psychiatric disorders will increase.
- Family stress will increase: suicides and homicides in the community will be attributed to the lack of community provision.
- The provision of private nursing homes will increase.
- Some people who would have been sent to mental hospitals will be sent to prison instead – with consequent management problems for the prison authorities.
- Mental hospitals will be utilized under other names – a process that Andrew Scull calls 'word-magic'. (Jones, 1998: 226)

Almost fourteen years after Jones's original predictions, all five of these appear to have been realized, especially in Britain, which I know better than the USA.[1]

Jenner (1998) acknowledged the 'truth' of Jones's observation but also noted that Jones had found exactly what she had gone looking for. More importantly, Jenner set the development in Italy in a paradigmatic context. When Galileo developed the telescope, in the seventeenth century, the majority of Italians wished to have nothing to do 'with this nonsense'. In Jenner's view, they would most probably have been too frightened to look into them. They might also have noted, had they been sufficiently aware, that Galileo really stole the idea from Copernicus and the Dutch lens grinders and wasn't so much original, as charismatic. The same may well have been true of Basaglia, whose ideas about reform and the whole complex business of caring for people 'in madness' had been around for a long time, before he brought his own charisma to bear on his 'reformation' of the Italian psychiatric scene.

FIXING OR UNDERSTANDING?

The notion of intersubjective reality fractures the fragile faith in subject–object duality so central to, and perhaps beloved of, classical psychiatry. Basaglia's re-socialization of the 'mad' fractured the inherent dualism between the 'sane' and the 'mad', the normal and the abnormal. Much of what has occurred in psychiatry, over the past decades, has involved 'breaks' with revered concepts, with an inevitable rise in separation anxiety.

We have paid some specific attention to language in this text, since this is – at least – the medium for our certainty/uncertainty. It might also be said – *pace* Saussure[2] – that language might only refer to itself: our uncertainty lies in the stating of our uncertainty. It is evident that the past 30 years have witnessed an increase in such statements of uncertainty, especially about the focus of psychiatry. We are aware that a range of terms has been employed, by different authors, in this text to refer to something, which once was called madness. What is not at all clear is whether or not everyone is addressing the same 'thing' or even group of 'things'.

Chung and Hill (1996) discussed the 'deeply rooted foundational-error-knowledge' from which the skills of classical psychiatrists are drawn. In their view such psychiatrists are unable to recognize themselves as holding such an error 'since their extensive psychiatric training and research leave no room for a revaluation of such a foundation . . . they only accept and take it for granted as if the foundation is the true knowledge' (1996: 329).

In Chung and Hill's view such 'thought-to-be-true knowledge' has become embedded within their cognitive structure. If one accepted that argument, one might conclude that such psychiatrists were 'cognitively impaired'. Such a view would not, commonly, be levelled, since the psychiatrist is the foundation of knowledge and, at the same time, is the agency who detects cognitive impairment in others, through use of his 'foundational knowledge'.

Bentall (1990) is one of the newer critics of classical psychiatric practice, who has argued that the construct validity of the classification – and diagnosis – of schizophrenia as a disease entity is problematic in the extreme. Given that delusions and hallucinations can occur in patients with affective disorders, and thought disorder can occur in manic patients, these 'symptoms' are not symptomatic – uniquely – of one condition, far less disease entity.

Kendell (1975) is one authority who is keen to redefine schizophrenia as a 'biological disadvantage', which results in an objectively verifiable impairment of functioning. This appears to be a plausible and reasonable view, until one examines the heterogeneity of psychosis further. Hearing 'voices' and seeing 'visions' or even feeling invisible 'presences', have been documented in schizophrenia, but are also evident in post-traumatic stress syndrome and bereavement reactions: auditory, visual and sensorimotor hallucinations. More importantly, apparently identical phenomena have been reported – for centuries by people experiencing mystical states. The experience of 'altered states' has yielded a strong body of evidence that so-called 'hallucinatory' experiences might be part of an expanded consciousness (Wilber, 1997) and even a 'spiritual emergence' (Grof, 1998). Perhaps the weakness of medical ambitions to define, once and for all, the root causes of such complex phenomena, lie in their efforts to isolate a single factor: reduction *ad absurdum*. It may well be the case that similar kinds of experience can occur in quite different human contexts. The challenge to psychiatry is to be able to tell the difference.

Of course the terminology of psychiatry is only part of a more complex project – the explanation of behaviour, emotion and consciousness. Traditionally, the psychiatric project has attempted to isolate the single, causative agent, responsible for the generation of (e.g.) hallucinations. Davey has written extensively of his experience of psychosis – using this as a vehicle to critique the increasingly popular stress-diathesis model of mental distress. He is patently uncomfortable with the idea that people who experience what is called psychosis are simply unable to cope with stressors in their environment, because of some inherent vulnerability, which is psychologically acquired. In Davey's view, such models of psychosis: 'neatly side-step an examination of the appalling circumstances in which people live here and now: it can perpetuate a host of personal and social injustices' (1996: 50).

Davey described the early stages of a serious depressive breakdown, when he lost a job that had been the core of his working and personal life for five years. He no longer had anything to talk about to people whom he knew very well, and he gradually retired from public life, seeing no future for himself.

> My psychiatrist was probably pondering on whether I was suffering from the depression of manic depression or the poverty of speech and affect typical of schizophrenic psychosis. I think he concluded the latter (because lithium didn't work it was not helpful to pigeonhole my problems as manic depression.) Retrospectively, I was suffering because the whole content had been emptied from my life. ... In retrospect it was obvious why I was suffering – but at the time I could not see it. Neither did my psychiatrist. (1996: 58)

Davey is, of course, talking about the meaning of his distress, rather than any isolated causative factor. It could be argued that his loss was the cause, but he might have emphasized that the loss was only significant in terms of who he was, and where he was – the whole of his experience – at that point in his life. It is in these very uncertainties that the intersubjective relationship, the social context of madness and personal meanings achieve some kind of holistic synthesis. Maybe Davey didn't want his despair fixed – perhaps he wanted it to be understood.

But if understanding is the name of the game, where should we turn for insight into that other place we call madness other than existing psychiatric texts? In the literary world, James Kelman (1993) in *How Late It Was, How Late*, describes the life world of Sammy. Sammy is disadvantaged in three health senses. He has lost his sight whilst being kept overnight in a police station after being beaten. He has a longstanding alcohol dependency, and is reacting emotionally to the loss of his partner and son. Through a riveting monologue we become steeped in the 'sense-making' of Sammy in relation to his encounters with the harsh world of downtown Glasgow. In the world of cinema, *Farewell My Concubine* (1993, directed by Chen Caige) charts the life history of a Chinese boy abandoned in his early years to the school of the Peking Opera. The film transmits to the viewer a sense of the fragility of the main character's existence and, ultimately, his suicide. These examples seem to point up the sterility of existing psychiatric understandings – usually of the order: she is depressed, he is manic, she is treatment-resistant – and invite us, the understanders, into a new realm of fiction stranger (more compelling) than fact.

DIRE PREDICTIONS

The notion of a creative exchange, between the psychiatric professional and the lay-patient, is in stark contrast to the modernist medical assumption that the patient is part of an external reality, an objective truth, open to exploration, and explication, by expert languages. Perhaps, most threatening of all, the notion of intersubjectivity and the alternative re-professionalization of psychiatric practice, imply chaotic exchanges.

When chaos theory emerged in the early 1960s it focused, mainly, on weather. At last we had a theoretical model for explaining the unreliability of long-term weather forecasting. The blushes of the forecasters, who had been expected to offer 'reliable' and 'accurate' predictions, but had even managed to miss the Great Storm of 1988, could be spared – with authority. Soon it became clear that unsystematic intrusions pervaded every corner of our lives: no known system – from the operation of gravity to the swinging of a pendulum – was, apparently, free from chaotic influence (Fernandez-Armesto, 1997). Chaos theory illuminated the breathtaking complexity of our world and, in principle, should have strengthened humankind's long search for 'the truth'. Ironically, in concert with several other chaotic movements in science, art and philosophy, chaos theory began to make its own contribution to the insidious erosion of certainty. The notion of a chaotic world, embedded within a chaotic universe, appeared to mirror some of the more tangible experiences, which confronted people: 'meaningless art and truthless thought' (Fernandez-Armesto, 1997: 187).

However, as we noted in our introductions to this text, all our concepts of 'the truth' have been social and linguistic constructions. If the truth is, indeed, 'out there' (apropos Mulder and Scully) then what is 'in here' is our perception, interpretation, framing, distortion and belief in that 'truth'. This betrays the most obvious of all truths – that the story of truth, like the story of art, science and every other human experience, is enacted – by actors. The key actors in our history, both ancient and contemporary are, of course, the victors: those elites who have erected monuments to themselves, or their kin, controlling the means of recording that history and holding 'the chroniclers, analysts and journalists in the palm of their patronage' (Fernandez-Armesto, 1997: 193). Within the context of contemporary psychiatry, this is as true of the editors of even the driest, academic journals. Their power involves determining who will receive the stamp of authority, through publication, and who will be consigned, along with their ideas, to the darkness of rejection. Academics will insist that this process is even-handed and impartial – focused on the selection of those papers which will take the scientific community closer towards 'quality' and 'truth'. Others might argue, even within the self-same academic communities, that there exists still too many opportunities for nepotism, favouritism and genuflection before politicized altars or obeisance to the religion of orthodoxy.

We emphasize this state of affairs as one of the timeless 'truths' concerning the manufacture of 'truth'. We are aware that some readers will read our editing of this text as merely another example of the same kind of partiality. We comfort ourselves, in this concluding epilogue, by reflecting on some of the 'chaotic stability' evident within the text. We have included arguments from the political right and left. We have illustrated the presumed strengths, as well as weaknesses, of diagnosis and classification. We have considered the negative influences of racism and the potential therapeutic power of compassion. In the spirit of chaos, all texts make some kind of dent on the reality of the emergent truth of history. This text may not be any less partial than others but, in our view, it has thrown its own chaotic net over a fair-sized stretch of the oceans of discourse. We hope also that we have dammed any threat of drowning in obfuscation.

When Foucault – that great leftist liberator – began to lose his own faith in any notion of an 'absolute truth', he had begun to appreciate that 'the truth' was no more than another instrument of oppression. Absolute truth appeared to differ little from any of the other oppressive 'truths': that women were inferior, that certain races were superior, and that those who bucked 'the system' most strongly could be defined as insane. This latter 'truth' found its most powerful and authoritative – yet local – form in Soviet psychiatry, where political dissidents were re-defined as mentally ill. Foucault's provisional conclusion was that some 'truths' were preferable to others; representing a regime, an ensemble of rules, which enjoyed a circular relation with systems of power that produced and sustained the same regime (Foucault, 1971).

THE SLIPPAGE OF TRUTH?

Just as chaos led, albeit unwittingly for the chaotic ideal, to more and more uncertainty, 'so Foucault's "system of exclusion" led to the post-modern nightmare where all utterances are of equal (little) value' (Fernandez-Armesto, 1997: p.194). In this nightmare liars have nothing to prove and defenders of truth have no case to demand of them. Fernandez-Armesto (1997) suggests, with the most trenchant irony, that we should all join the voiceless, revel in illiteracy and abandon language!

Examples of the 'slippage of truth' in the contemporary world are all around us. Perhaps, however, psychiatry clings to a more solid, reliable, truth about people, their experience, and our experience of them as 'others'. The following examples may illustrate one dimension of the 'preferability' of truth, addressed by Foucault, and may show how power – and powerlessness – continues to be the hallmark of madness.

A young woman, deemed by public consensus to be 'slim and attractive', disports herself on a television chat show in an apparently drunken state. She swears at the host and abuses the other guests. In the middle of the proceedings, she abandons the stage. The tale of the talk show makes many headlines the following day and the woman's agent uses the story to publicize further her art exhibition. The 'show' features, among other 'works' a tent, inside of which she has sewn the names of all the people she has slept with during her (short) life. In an interview at her studio at 9.30 in the morning a week later, the young woman invites the interviewer to join her in a 'few cans of lager', as she deliberates whether or not she should have a baby by artificial insemination.

A different woman, unkindly referred to as having a 'careworn appearance', often gets drunk and abusive and 'emotional' in public. Recently, she publicly displayed the name of a married man who had slept with her, then returned to his long-suffering wife. She becomes distressed and seeks organized (social) attention, is diagnosed as a 'personality disorder', threatened with detention under the Mental Health Act, and is advised that perhaps she should consider surrendering her children to a care agency.

A middle-aged man is found to have been having sex with one of his staff while at work. Because of his position he faces an obscure charge of political impropriety. His lawyer denies that his client 'actually' had sexual intercourse, but admits that the woman – who was an unpaid and low-ranking member of the office staff – did offer sexual 'favours' which were accepted by the man. The story is reported world-wide on the Internet and a famous playwright compares the 'hounding' of the man, for what is no more than 'private sexual activity', to the Salem witch hunts and subsequent trials.

Another middle-aged man is 'found' to have been masturbating in a toilet at the day care service he attends. The man is characterized as having a 'long term mental health problem'. He has been in and out of care for several years. The person who 'found' him was a care officer. The event was not reported to the papers, but was discussed, intensively at a case conference, where various 'options' – ranging from exclusion from the day care service, to prescription of medication – were discussed. The man was not present and was not represented by a lawyer.

As this book is written, we are only months away from the turn of the Millennium, an event in the Christian calendar, which is trumpeted more, perhaps, by materialists, who want to build domes to signify human progress, or some such other tangible symbol. Increasingly, we live in a Mickey Mouse world in which confusion is treated as 'good', the social world whirring on its inane axis. Pluralism has already become stuck in pastiche and, if people increasingly stop believing in 'something', it is not – as Fernandez-Armesto observed, 'to begin believing in nothing'. Despite predictions to the contrary, nihilism has not returned. Indeed, the situation might even be classed as worse than nihilism: people have begun to 'believe in anything'. Crackpot cults prosper, manipulative sects thrive, discredited superstitions revive (Fernandez-Armesto, 1997).

So, is the search for truth over and do we have to settle for truthless truths? Wilber may come to our aid when he notes that:

> Truth is radically formless, spaceless and timeless, encompassing all space and time but limited to none. ... We cannot make a statement about the whole of Reality [sic], because any conceivable statement is itself merely part of that Reality, and thus the perennial philosophy, as a direct insight-union with that reality itself, could never be adequately captured in any set of doctrines or ideas, all of which are partial, finite, and limited. Radical truth can be shown (in contemplative awareness) but never exhaustively said (in discursive language). (Wilber, 1997: 59)

This may be the nettle that psychiatry needs to grasp (or ungrasp), which signifies the uncertainties, not only of the search for truth, but also for meaning, and all the other altruistic and territorial ambitions of the human project.

NOTES

1 Personal contacts and experience of the USA and Australia and New Zealand suggest a similar picture there.
2 In Saussure's view no language could yield formulations assuredly true of anything except its own terms. Meaning would, in his view, always be incomplete, representing the unbridgeable chasm between any 'term' and its 'referent'. Such a chasm did not apply, of course, between a term and itself, or a sentence and what it was supposed to be about. In Hofstader's view, language was entangled, inextricably, in trammels of 'strange loopiness' (Hofstader, 1980).
3 Those who attempt to uncover and explain the underlying essence and the causative laws and principles that govern the thoughts and behaviour of the mad (Chung and Hill, 1996: 324).

REFERENCES

Barker, P. (1999) *The Philosophy and Practice of Psychiatric Nursing*. London: Churchill Livingstone.

Bentall, R.P. (1990) *Reconstructing Schizophrenia*. London: Methuen.

Cawley, R.H. (1993) Psychiatry is more than a science. *British Journal of Psychiatry*, **162**: 154–60.

Chung, M.C. and Hill, R.G. (1996) The relevance of Plato's Thaetetus in some classical and antipsychiatrist's debates. *Changes*, **14**(4): 324–9.

Davey, B. (1996) Upbringing and psychosis. *Changes*, **14**(1): 50–63.

Evans, F.B. (1996) *Harry Stack Sullivan: Interpersonal Theory and Psychotherapy*. London: Routledge.

Fernandez-Armesto, F. (1997) *Truth: a History*. London: Bantam Press.

Grof, S. (1998) *The Cosmic Game: Explorations in the Frontiers of Human Consciousness*. Dublin: Newleaf.

Hofstader, D. (1980) Gödel, Escher, Bach: an Eternal Golden Braid. Harmondsworth: Penguin.

Jenner, H.S. (1998) Seeing the alternatives. Changes, **16**(3): 229–33.

Jones, K. (1998) Mid-line crisis. *Changes*, **16**(3): 223–38.

Kelman, J. (1993) *How Late It was, How Late*. London: Secker and Warburg.

Kendell, R.E. (1975) *The Role of Diagnosis in Psychiatry*. Oxford: Blackwell Scientific Publications.

Kotowicz, Z. (1996) *R.D. Laing and the Paths of Anti-psychiatry*. London: Routledge.

Rogers, A., Pilgrim, D. and Lacey, R. (1993) *Experiencing Psychiatry: Users' Views of Services*. London: MIND/Macmillan.

Sullivan, H.S. (1953) *The Interpersonal Theory of Psychiatry*. New York: W.W. Norton & Company.

Thomas, P. (1997) *The Dialectics of Schizophrenia*. London: Free Association Books.

Wilber, K. (1997) *The Eye of the Spirit: an Integral Vision for a World Gone Slightly Mad*. London: Shambhala.

Zohar, D. (1991) *The Quantum Self*. London: Flamingo/Harper Collins.

Index